GW00775826

The 30-Minute Mediterranean diet

111 best-ever simple recipes for your health and vitality

By

Slavka Bodic

Please sign up for free Balkan and Mediterranean recipes:
www.balkanfood.org

Table Of Contents

Lunch Recipes_____ 60

Why The Mediterranean Diet?

Unlike conventional diets, the Mediterranean diet doesn't restrict you to a daily allotment of calories, fat, or sodium. Instead, it's about what you're eating, from heart-healthy unsaturated fats to satiating, high-fibre foods. Recipes maximize flavour and nutrition to create balanced plates that marry whole grains with vegetables, lean proteins, and more. On top of all of this deliciously nutritious eating, make sure to work physical activity into your day, especially if you have a desk job.

Based on Mediterranean diet principles, it is easy to change healthy eating habits and really lose weight in a sustainable way. A diet is not only "stop eating carbs" and "try the newest weight loss pill"—because at the end, we are all frustrated with results. No, you will not become a supermodel after two weeks, but if you accept principles of the Mediterranean diet (which should include some physical activity if possible), you will solve a problem in the long run. Moreover, I you probably already know that world-leading cardiologists recommend this diet to all their patients. Yes, people in and around the Mediterranean region have much lower rates of heart diseases than those living in other parts of the world.

The Greek life philosophy *everything in moderation* should become your new mantra.

Slavka Bodic

Why This Book (And Not Another One)?

Yes, I know. You already read many blogs on the Mediterranean diet and probably bought some book about it—maybe some fancy cookbook with many nice photos or the ones with photos of Greek islands. However, you need to choose between nice photos and a healthier life. I read so many e-cookbooks, especially the ones focused on Mediterranean diet, and I always find three problems.

Firstly, meals are complicated to prepare, even for someone from the region, like me. Maybe the idea is to spend the whole day in the kitchen and lose your weight while preparing these meals. However, I am not saying that meals in these cookbooks are not delicious or healthy. On the contrary, they are quite good, but you need to be a chef to prepare the majority of them.

Secondly, some of these recipes are expensive to prepare. I saw comments where people say that they need 300-400 USD to prepare lunch: or dinner from some cookbooks. My guess is that this is not acceptable for the majority of readers. Moreover, such expensive dishes have nothing to do with the Mediterranean region. On the contrary, meals in that part of the world are cheap, but tasty. This should be the case for recipes suggested for this diet.

Thirdly, almost every diet cookbook is extremely rigid, which means no dessert, no chocolate, and no cheating day. If you strictly follow the rules, you will probably be thinking about the food you want to eat (except when you are preparing costly 120-minute meals). Finally, when you are stressed or simply cannot stand anymore, you will eat some ice cream, chocolate or any food you like. According to all books, this will destroy what you achieved in previous weeks or months. Your diet should change your eating habits in a sustainable way that will result in a better and happier life, not obsessing over the of bread or dessert that you ate during lunch: with a friend.

In this cookbook, I promise you will find:

- Simple meals that you can cook within 30 minutes.
- Affordable (or better– cheap) dishes that could be prepared with several ingredients. Of course, I am not counting regular ones as salt, paper, milk, water, etc.
- Tasty recipes that you will like to eat. Yes, you can enjoy food during your diet.
- Losing weight in a sustainable way that will not make you hungry, depressive, or nervous.

Yes, I also promise that ice cream once in couple of weeks is not a tragedy.

Key Principles Of The Mediterranean Diet

Take a look into Mediterranean diet pyramid (or triangle).

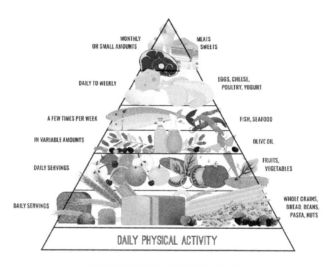

MONTHLY OR SMALL AMOUNTS — MEATS SWEETS

DAILY TO WEEKLY — EGGS, CHEESE, POULTRY, YOGURT

A FEW TIMES PER WEEK — FISH, SEAFOOD

IN VARIABLE AMOUNTS — OLIVE OIL

DAILY SERVINGS — FRUITS, VEGETABLES

DAILY SERVINGS — WHOLE GRAINS, BREAD, BEANS, PASTA, NUTS

DAILY PHYSICAL ACTIVITY

MEDITERRANEAN DIET

As you can see, the base of the pyramid/triangle consists of food that should be eaten in the largest amounts (whole grains, vegetables, nuts, fruits, legumes, beans, seeds, herbs). Eat it a lot, daily. Some physical activity every day is a must. No, you don't need to do heavy lifting at the local gym, but a 30 min. daily walk will help.

The next level (2-3 a week) is reserved for fish and seafood that should be eaten 3 times a week. They will provide you with Omega-3 essential fatty acids. Poultry, eggs, and cheese are the third level, and you should consume them once a week. However, it is not a catastrophe if you eat a chicken meal twice during the week.

At the end, red meat, processed food and sweets are on the top of the pyramid and they should be consumed minimally, or not at all.

Drinking water is a must.

Additional key principles

- At least once a week, build meals around beans, whole grains, and vegetables, and heighten the flavor with fragrant herbs and spices—fully without meat.
- Include sources of healthy fats in daily meals, especially extra-virgin olive oil, nuts, olives, and avocados. The American Heart Association recommends using healthy cooking oils such as canola, peanut, and safflower.
- Include whole grains that are naturally rich with many important nutrients.
- Instead of daily ice cream or cookies, save sweets for special occasion once every ten days. Choose from a wide range of delicious fresh fruits — from apples and oranges to pomegranates, grapes, and strawberries.
- Herbs and spices make food tasty and are also rich in health-promoting substances. Season your meals with herbs and spices rather than salt.
- Have a glass of wine at dinner. If you don't drink alcohol, purple grape juice may be an alternative to wine.

Summary Of The Diet

Frequent:

Vegetables: From a simple plate of sliced fresh tomatoes drizzled with olive oil and feta cheese, to salads, garlicky greens, soups and stews, healthy pizzas, or oven-roasted medleys, vegetables are vitally important. Whether raw, grilled, steamed, sautéed, roasted, or pickled, vegetables should be on your plate every meal.

Whole grains: A 2015 study in JAMA Internal Medicine linked whole grains and lower mortality—especially from chronic diseases such as cardiovascular disease and type-2 diabetes. Common whole grains include brown rice and oats, while ancient grains such as quinoa, amaranth, farro, buckwheat, and bulgur pack the added perk of being gluten-free. Their fuller taste and extra fiber keep you satisfied for hours.

Water, physical activity, and wine (once a day). Coffee and tea are also completely acceptable, but you should avoid sugar-sweetened beverages and fruit juices, which are very high in sugar.

Frequent but moderate:

Fish and seafood three times a week: Fish such as tuna, herring, salmon, and sardines are rich in omega-3 fatty acids, and shellfish including mussels, oysters, and clams have similar benefits for brain and heart health. Poultry, eggs and cheese should be limited to once a week.

Avoid:

Sweets, red meat and processed food.

As I mentioned above, you can eat this kind of food, but as an exception. I also believe that you should have "cheat meal" once a month and I include several delicious meals in this book as a suggestion for that day. A more detailed list of food and ingredients to avoid is the following:

- Trans fats: Found in margarine and various processed foods
- Added sugar: Soda, candies, ice cream, table sugar, etc.
- Refined grains: White bread, pasta made with refined wheat, etc.
- Highly processed foods: Anything labeled "low-fat" or "diet", or which looks like it was made in a factory
- Refined oils: Soybean oil, cottonseed oil etc. (please note that experts disagree if canola oil should be used or not)
- Processed meat: Processed sausages, hot dogs, etc.

You must read food labels carefully if you want to avoid the unhealthy ingredients listed above.

Questions and Myths

Is it expensive?

If you plan properly, you will buy only what you need during the week. Many ingredients can be bought in bulk. Since you should buy a lot of vegetables and fruits, focus on the ones that are in season in order to get the best prices. Fresh fish fillets might be expensive to buy, so you can buy frozen supplement fish. The only difference is olive oil or seed oils that are a bit more expensive. In general, this diet is not expensive, and I wrote this book to present the most affordable recipes.

Mediterranean diet is a fad diet

Is it popular? Yes, very popular in the Mediterranean region. Also, it is very popular among cardiologists and other doctors. However, it is not one of those fashionably diets for this session.

How it is possible to have a diet but eating all types of food?

It is possible, because it is not natural to fully exclude all kinds of food. The point is to limit the weekly amount of some types of food and to maximize healthy choices.

Is it hard to follow?

Well, if you hate vegetables and fruits and adore red meat, it could be hard for you at the beginning. However, from the experience of my friends (and my personal experience), things are much better after week or two.

What are the benefits of Mediterranean diet?

According to researchers, there are many benefits of this diet, but the key ones that you will find in every blog, book or website are the following:

- Reduces risk of type II diabetes, depression, anxiety, and certain type of cancers
- Reduces body fat, high blood pressure and bad cholesterol (LDL)
- Reduces risk of death from heart disease by 72%
- Increases good cholesterol (HDL) and longevity
- Improves mental function, mood, and the look of your skin
- Safeguards against Alzheimer's and Parkinson's diseases

Your Plan: Adopting the Mediterranean Lifestyle

Since you are already familiar with Mediterranean pyramid, it is quite easy to have idea what you should eat and what to avoid. Despite the fact that diet is "Mediterranean", you can eat Mexican, Japanese, Indian or Balkan food (the Balkan region partly overlaps with the Mediterranean). In my already published book "Ultimate BALKAN cookbook: TOP 35 Balkan dishes that you can prepare right now", you can find many tasty traditional recipes both for every day and for your "cheat day". At the end of this book, I added three dishes from that book that I fully recommend. They are tasty, inexpensive, and easy to prepare.

You can stick to many different plans if you will start with Mediterranean diet. Many of them are presented in different blogs, websites, and books. I will present my suggestion in this book. However, the key is to eat small but frequent meals. You should not skip any meal since that may affect your blood sugar level. Yes, snacks are also fully acceptable (no, ice creams, chocolate or cookies are not snacks).

I know that you are probably already obsessed with calories and that you might read number of calories when shopping in the market. However, the Mediterranean diet is not about calories. Of course, you must take as few calories as possible, but depriving your body of needed nutrition will increase level of cortisol, a stress hormone. Cortisol will negatively affect your metabolism, while fat will be stored in hips, thighs, and abdomen as a result of it.

Preparation

Apart from informing your family and minimizing the amount of cookies around you, it is good to start with stocking your kitchen for the diet:

Spices: oregano, powdered garlic, onion powder, curry (not typical Mediterranean, but you will use it), basil, mint, red chili flakes. You probably have salt and black paper already.
Sweetener: Stevia and honey are the key, but you can use maple syrup and agave nectar as well.

Rice: brown—wild and basmati

Bread: Plain croutons, sprouted bread. etc.

Oil: Extra virgin olive, olive, coconut

Vinegar: Red, apple cider, balsamic, white

Seeds and walnuts: sunflower seeds, sesame seeds, walnuts, cashew nuts, almonds

Whole wheat pasta

Wine (red)

Canned soups if you are in hurry and dark chocolate (70% cocoa) if you are in a crisis

Snacks: organic salsa, hummus, soy chips, unsalted crackers, plain rice cakes

Vegetables, fruits, fish/seafood and poultry are not in this list, since you should buy them based on your weekly or daily plan.

Once when you done and ready to start, calculate how many calories you will consume (or you are already taking). It should be less than 1300 calories for woman and less than 1950 for man. If you want to eat more, you can do this, but physical activity must be increased accordingly. If you fully stick to plan and recipes, you can lose 2 lbs weekly without stress and hunger.

Advices from My Experience That Can Help You To Succeed

Enjoy slow

I love watching TV and I often would eat in front of the TV, but I realized that I was not enjoying or even remembering parts of the meal. Attention was on television and not on the food. If you are doing the same, you are probably swallowing food in one bite. More than a diet, the Mediterranean diet is a lifestyle that teaches you to enjoy all the flavours of the food you eat. Eat slowly, take your time, taste, and enjoy. Eating slow will also tune your body with the food you eat. Enjoying your meals will even make you eat until you are just satisfied and prevent overeating.

Prepare new recipes for the loved ones

As I already mentioned, the Mediterranean diet is fully based on the principles of enjoyment and pleasure. As much as possible, eat with family and friends. Prepare these and other recipes for them. The happy company of others makes the food taste even better, and the laughter you share makes life even better. Yes, also criticize me and others if some recipes are not that nice. After some time, you and your family will modify some of these recipes and use some improved version.

Eggs are not enemies

I used to be scared about eating eggs, thinking that they are full of calories and that I should fully avoid them if I want to lose my weight. Wrong! Eggs are excellent sources of high-quality protein and are valuable for vegetarians and people who do not eat meat. Be sure to follow the recommended portions and frequency, but never exclude eggs.

Healthy Lifestyle is Possible

My physical activity was limited to cooking and shopping. Walking or anything else was an exception, while swimming was reserved for holiday time. After several different diets, I realize that overall health not only depends on a healthy eating habit. Together, with the Mediterranean diet, I start walking a lot. Gym and heavy exercise was not good enough for me, but I started walking more and more every day. Taking the stairs instead of the elevator is something what we all can do. Of course, running, aerobics, and other strenuous exercises is the best option.

Whole-Grain Food

One of my biggest problems with the Mediterranean diet was adjusting to whole-wheat and whole grain. As I already mention, moderate steps are they key. I slowly replaced refined grain products with whole-grain ones. If you have a similar problem, try mixing whole-grains with refined grained, half white and half whole-wheat. When your body has adjusted, then you can switch to whole-wheat and whole-grain completely.

Moderation

I am not moderate in many things. Since I was born and raised in the Balkans (many countries belong both to the Balkans and Mediterranean), that influences my temperament regarding both food and life in general. I tried many diets, and all of them involved eliminating certain foods. I was successful and strict for four weeks, felt bad another four, and then gave up. The Mediterranean diet is the first diet that accommodates a wide range of drinks and food. The message is to eat moderately and wisely, and that is why it works for me fully. I enjoy a slice of cake, a couple of slices of steak, wine, and much more. However, you really need to follow the recommended food frequency and portion size.

Hydrate

The body is made up of 70 percent water, and proper hydration is essential to maintain energy levels, health, and well-being. I used to drink only several glasses of water a day. However, after some tests, I realized that this level of dehydration affect processes in my body. The truth is that differences in metabolic rates, activity levels, and body type mean that some people need more water than others, but you should really try to drink as much water as possible.

Suggested Weekly Menu
Option 1

Monday

Breakfast: Omelette
Lunch: Black bean salad
Snack: Hummus with vegetables
Dinner: Chicken casserole

Tuesday

Breakfast: Greek yogurt with strawberries and oats
Lunch: Grilled salmon
Snack: Grilled fruit
Dinner: Pasta with salad

Wednesday

Breakfast: Fruit & yogurt smoothie
Lunch: Beans and rice
Snack: Two boiled eggs
Dinner: Cabbage apple slaw with baked fish

Thursday

Breakfast: Couscous
Lunch: Chickpea and bean soup

Snack: Fruit and nut bar
Dinner: Turkey or chicken dish

Friday

Breakfast: Omelette
Lunch: Black bean salad
Snack: Hummus with vegetables
Dinner: Chicken casserole

Saturday

Breakfast: Frittata
Lunch: Vegetable pasta
Snack: Fruit yogurt
Dinner: Pizza (but healthy one)

Sunday

Breakfast: Buckwheat pancakes
Lunch: Black bean salad
Snack: Wholegrain toast
Dinner: Grilled fish (or seafood) with brown rice

Suggested Weekly Many Option 2

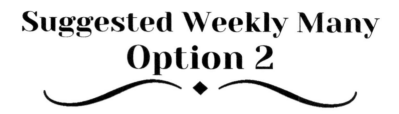

Monday

Breakfast: Eggs with vegetables
Lunch: Whole-grain sandwich with vegetables
Snack: Crackers with cheese
Dinner: A tuna salad, dressed in olive oil

Tuesday

Breakfast: Oatmeal with raisins
Lunch: Leftover tuna salad from the night before or seafood
Snack: Two boiled eggs
Dinner: Salad with tomatoes, olives and feta cheese

Wednesday

Breakfast: Omelet with veggies, tomatoes and onions
Lunch: Whole-grain sandwich, with cheese and fresh vegetables
Snack: Hummus with vegetables
Dinner: Broiled salmon, served with brown rice and vegetables

Thursday

Breakfast: Yogurt with sliced fruits and nuts
Lunch: Grilled chicken

Snack: Tzatziki dip with pita bread
Dinner: Mediterranean lasagna

Friday

Breakfast: Eggs and vegetables, fried in olive oil
Lunch: Greek yogurt with strawberries or other fruits, oats and nuts
Snack: Fruit and nut bar
Dinner: Grilled lamb, with salad and baked potato

Saturday

Breakfast: Oatmeal with raisins, nuts and an apple
Lunch: Whole-grain sandwich with vegetables
Snack: Chocolate (dark one with at least 70% cocoa)
Dinner: Mediterranean pizza (healthy one)

Sunday

Breakfast: Omelette with veggies and olives
Lunch: Grilled salmon or vegetable wrap
Snack: Fruits
Dinner: Grilled chicken, with vegetables and a potato

Suggested Weekly Many Option 3

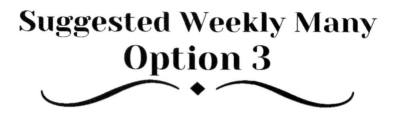

Monday

Breakfast: Mediterranean toast
Lunch: Tabouli
Snack: Fig smoothie with cinnamon
Dinner: Chicken kebab

Tuesday

Breakfast: Shakshouka
Lunch: Cretan pasta with salmon
Snack: Banana and peanuts yogurt
Dinner: Grilled salad nachos

Wednesday

Breakfast: Oatmeal with honey roasted plums
Lunch: Grilled shrimp salad with dill dressing
Snack: Greek dip
Dinner: Grilled salmon with vegetables

Thursday

Breakfast: Italian tofu scramble
Lunch: Avocado salad with radish and cucumber

Snack: Greek cucumber roll ups
Dinner: Mediterranean edamame toss

Friday

Breakfast: Greek fluffy pancakes
Lunch: Grilled salmon salad with yogurt
Snack: Salmon and goat cheese bites
Dinner: Spanish salmon tacos

Saturday

Breakfast: Greek quinoa breakfast bowl
Lunch: Tuna pasta
Snack: Feta, hummus and bell pepper crackers
Dinner: Italian tilapia

Sunday

Breakfast: Mediterranean frittata
Lunch: Roasted vegetable kebab
Snack: Fruit and nut snack mix
Dinner: Tuna wraps

Breakfast Recipes

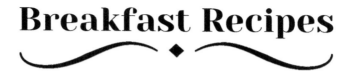

Strawberry Smoothie

Preparation time: 5 minutes

Ingredients
- 1 juicy peach
- ½ cup Greek yogurt or plain yogurt
- 1 small banana
- ⅔ cup hulled strawberries
- 1 tsp flaxseeds

Preparation
Cut the peach in half, remove the pit and cube the pulp. Add all ingredients to a food processor. Blitz until the ingredients are combined. Serve immediately, or chill before serving.

Fig & Pistachio & Avocado Smoothie

Preparation time: 8 minutes

Ingredients
4 fresh figs
½ cup shelled pistachios
2 cup milk
1 avocado, pit removed
2 bananas
½ teaspoon cinnamon
1 teaspoon vanilla
2 cup milk
1 avocado, pit removed
2 bananas
½ teaspoon cinnamon
1 teaspoon vanilla extract

Preparation
In a blender, combine all ingredients and blend until smooth and creamy.

Honeyed Yogurt with figs & Pistachio

Preparation time: 9 minutes

Ingredients
1½ cups plain Greek yogurt
2 tablespoons honey
1 teaspoon cinnamon
4 quartered figs
¼ cup pistachios
1 teaspoon cinnamon
4 quartered figs
¼ cup crushed pistachios

Preparation
In a bowl, mix together yogurt, honey and cinnamon. Divide sweetened yogurt between glasses and top with figs and pistachios.

Mediterranean scrambled eggs with feta, spinach and tomato

Preparation time: 5 minutes

Ingredients
1 tablespoon vegetable oil
1/3 cup tomato, diced and seeded (roughly 1/2 a medium tomato)
1 cup baby spinach
3 eggs
2 tablespoons feta cheese, cubed
salt and pepper to taste

Preparation
Heat oil in a frying pan on medium heat. Sauté the tomatoes and spinach until the spinach is wilted. Add all the eggs and mix to scramble. After 30-40 seconds, add the feta cheese. Continue to cook until the egg is cooked to your preference. Season with salt and pepper.

Mediterranean morning egg salad

Preparation time: 5 minutes (if you already have hardboiled eggs)

Ingredients
8 hardboiled eggs
1/2 cup sun-dried tomatoes, drained of excess oil and chopped
1/2 cup finely chopped red onion
1/2 chopped cucumber
1/4 cup chopped olives
1/2 cup plain Greek yogurt
splash of lemon juice
1 1/2 teaspoon of oregano
1/4 teaspoon of cumin
1/2 teaspoon of sea salt
freshly ground black pepper

Preparation
Chop up your hardboiled eggs and place them in a bowl. Add in sun-dried tomatoes, red onion, cucumber, and olives. Stir in Greek yogurt, lemon juice, and spices. Will keep for up to five days in the fridge.

Greek Quinoa Breakfast Bowl

Preparation time: 27 minutes

Ingredients (for six servings)
12 eggs
¼ cup plain Greek yogurt
1 teaspoon onion powder
1 teaspoon granulated garlic
½ teaspoon salt
½ teaspoon pepper
1 teaspoon olive oil
1 (5-ounce) bag baby spinach
1 pint cherry tomatoes, halved
1 cup feta cheese
2 cups cooked quinoa

Preparation
In a large bowl whisk together eggs, Greek yogurt, onion powder, granulated garlic, salt, and pepper. Set aside. In a large skillet heat olive oil and add spinach. Cook spinach until it is slightly wilted, 4 minutes.

Add in cherry tomatoes and cook until tomatoes are softened, no more than 4 minutes. Stir in egg mixture and cook until the eggs are set, about 8 minutes. Stir the eggs as they cook so they turn out scrambled. Once the eggs are set stir in the feta and quinoa and cook until heated through. Serve hot. Will keep for up to six days in the fridge. Heat in a microwave.

Mediterranean Frittata

Preparation time: 24 minutes

Ingredients (for five servings)
6 eggs
1/4 cup crumbled feta
1/2 cup milk or cream
1/2 cup diced tomatoes
1/4 cup chopped Kalamata olives
1/4 cup chopped Spanish olives
1 teaspoon salt
1 teaspoon oregano
1/2 teaspoon pepper

Preparation
Preheat oven to 400 degrees. Grease 8-inch pie pan or quiche dish. Whisk up all eggs and milk together until well blended. Add in remaining ingredients and mix well. Bake for no more than 20 minutes or until eggs are set.

Shakshouka

Preparation time: 27 minutes

Ingredients
4 eggs
1 sliced onion
1 tablespoon of chopped parsley
2 sliced red bell peppers
2 chopped garlic cloves
1.15 oz can chopped tomatoes
1 teaspoon of sugar
3/4 teaspoon of spicy harissa
2 tablespoons olive oil
Salt and pepper to taste

Preparation
Heat the oil in a heavy skillet (like cast iron). Add onions and peppers and cook them until soft for about 4-5 minutes, stirring occasionally. After that, add garlic and cook for another minute. Add tomatoes, sugar and harissa and cook for about 7 minutes. Season with salt and pepper and add more harissa if you want more spice.

With wooden spoon, make 4 indentations in the mixture and add egg in each of them.
Cover the pot and cook until the egg whites are just set. In total, cooking time should not be more than 20 minutes. Sprinkle with fresh parsley and serve immediately with pita bread or crusty bread.

Mediterranean toast

Preparation time: 3 minutes

Ingredients
1 slice whole wheat or multi-grain bread
1/4 mashed avocado
1 sliced hard-boiled egg
1 tablespoon of roasted red pepper hummus
3 sliced grape/cherry tomatoes
3 sliced Greek olives
1 1/2 teaspoon reduced fat crumbled feta cheese

Preparation
Toast the slice of bread and top it with the 1 teaspoon of hummus, and 1/4 mashed avocado. Add the sliced cherry tomatoes and olives, followed by the sliced hardboiled egg and feta. Add salt and pepper to taste.

Italian cappuccino muffins

Preparation time: 27 minutes

Ingredients (12 servings)
2 cups of all-purpose flour
1 egg
½ cup brown sugar
½ cup cream
1 cup strong espresso or very strong brewed coffee
1 tablespoon of baking powder
Powdered sugar to garnish (try to avoid too much sugar)
Pinch of salt

Preparation
Preheat oven to 350 F and brush the muffin pan with butter. Add flour, baking powder, and salt to a bowl and mix together. Make a hole in the middle of the flour and add sugar. Beat egg and cream with a hand mixer. Add the egg & cream mixture, as well as the coffee into the flour. Beat well with the hand mixer.

Pour the muffin mix into the muffin pan. Bake for about 20 minutes. To ensure they are fully cooked, poke with a knife. If the knife comes out dry, they are ready, if not, bake more. Allow the muffins to cool and then decorate with powdered sugar.

Avocado toast with salmon

Preparation time: 8 minutes

Ingredients (for two servings)
2 ounces smoked salmon, thinly sliced
1 ripe avocado
10 capers
4-5 small slices of bread
A few thin slices of red onion
Juice of ½ lemon
A few small stems fresh dill
Dash of salt

Preparation
Cut avocado in half, remove pit. Scoop out flesh and mash with a dash of salt and lemon juice. Toast bread. Spread avocado on toast. Top with capers. Top avocado and capers with a slice or two of smoked salmon and then with dill and red onion slices. Serve immediately (not suitable for keeping in the fridge).

Syrian Ful Medames

Preparation time: 19 minutes

Ingredients (for two servings)
1 15 oz can fava beans
1/4 red onion, diced
1/2 tablespoon cumin
1 diced tomato
3 tablespoon tahini
Juice of 1 lemon
Handful of fresh chopped parley
Extra virgin olive oil

Preparation
Put the fava beans with the liquid in a small saucepan on high heat. Bring to a boil, add cumin, salt, pepper, and lower to medium heat. Cook 9-10 minutes, stirring often. Remove from heat. Mash beans with a fork to desired consistency. Whisk together tahini and lemon juice. Add to fava beans. Mix well.

Transfer the beans to a serving bowl. Top liberally with fresh chopped parsley, diced tomato, diced onion, and a drizzle of extra virgin olive oil.

Stewed Prunes with Greek Yogurt

Preparation time: 28 minutes

Ingredients
1 cup pitted prunes
1 teaspoon honey
1 thin slice lemon with rind
1 cup plain Greek yogurt
2 cups water
½ teaspoon cinnamon

Preparation
Add all stewed prune ingredients to a small pot. Bring to a boil and then simmer on a low boil, uncovered, for 19-20 minutes. Continue to simmer, covered, for 10 more minutes. Fill two bowls with ½ cup of yogurt each. Make a well in the yogurt and then add prunes and syrup. Sprinkle cinnamon on top. Add half lemon slice from prunes for garnish.

Lime, pineapple and orange smoothie

Preparation time: 4 minutes

Ingredients
2 oranges
1 cup of pineapple chunks
1 lime
1/2 cup vanilla yogurt

Preparation
Puree all ingredients in a blender on the high setting. Garnish with pineapple wedges, orange slices or mint.

Mango and strawberry smoothie

Preparation time: 10 minutes

Ingredients (for two servings)
1/2 cup frozen strawberries
1 banana
1/2 cup frozen mango
1/4 cup almond milk (or soy or cow)
1/2 cup Greek yogurt
1/4 teaspoon turmeric
1/4 teaspoon ginger
1 tablespoon honey

Preparation
Blend all ingredients in blender until smooth.

Savory Breakfast Polenta with Eggs, Spinach and Onions

Preparation time: 20 minutes

Ingredients (for two servings)
2 eggs
1/2 cup instant polenta
1 cup whole milk (or milk of your choice)
handful of spinach, stems removed
1/2 teaspoon salt
1 teaspoon butter
2 tablespoons Parmesan cheese
1 onion, sliced into thin rounds
1 teaspoon extra virgin olive oil
1 minced clove garlic
1 cup water
1/2 teaspoon balsamic vinegar

Preparation
Bring milk, water, salt, and butter to a boil, stirring often so milk doesn't scald. On low heat, add polenta, stirring continuously. Add more water depending on desired creaminess. Take off heat and add Parmesan cheese. Heat olive oil in a skillet. Add onions and sauté for about 3 minutes or until soft. Add spinach. Cook until spinach is wilted. Add garlic and balsamic vinegar. Mix well. Remove spinach and onions with a slotted spoon or tongs. Fry eggs in remaining liquid. Add salt and pepper to taste. Spread half of polenta on each plate. Spoon on half of spinach/egg mixture and then top with an egg.

Red Pepper Tapenade on Toast

Preparation time: 27 minutes

Ingredients (for five servings)
1/2 cup pitted Kalamata olives
1 tablespoon lemon juice
1 lb. of fresh mozzarella, thinly sliced
1 tablespoon capers
1 cup roasted red peppers
2 tablespoon chopped cilantro
6 pieces of sourdough toasted bread
1 teaspoon ground cumin
1/2 teaspoon Aleppo pepper
1/2 teaspoon garlic powder
1/2 teaspoon onion powder
1/4 teaspoon cardamom
1/4 cup extra virgin olive oil
pepper to taste

Preparation
Place Kalamata olives, olive oil, lemon juice, capers, cumin, Aleppo pepper, garlic powder, onion powder, cardamom and pepper in food processor. Process until ingredients are chopped finely, but not pureed.

Place olive mix in a bowl. Add roasted red peppers to food processor and process until chopped. Add cilantro and process until finely chopped. Mix roasted red pepper mix in with olive mix. Cut toasted bread slices in half and layer each piece of toast with sliced mozzarella then add a large dollop of tapenade.

Tomato and Zucchini Frittata

Preparation time: 27 minutes

Ingredients (for five servings)
8 eggs
1 small thinly sliced lengthwise zucchini
½ cup halved cherry tomatoes
2 ounces bite-size fresh mozzarella balls
1/3 cup coarsely chopped walnuts
¼ teaspoon salt
¼ teaspoon crushed red pepper
1 tablespoon olive oil

Preparation
Preheat broiler. In a medium bowl whisk together eggs and crushed red pepper. Add salt. Heat olive oil in a 10-inch oven-going skillet over medium-high heat. Layer zucchini slices on bottom of skillet in an even layer. Cook for 3 minutes, turning once. Top with prepared cherry tomatoes.

Pour egg mixture over vegetables in skillet. Top with mozzarella balls and chopped walnuts. Cook over medium heat up to 5 minutes or until sides begin to set, lifting with a spatula to allow the uncooked portion to run underneath. Broil 4 inches from the heat up to 3 minutes more or until set. Cut into wedges to serve.

Ham and eggs cups

Preparation time: 22 minutes

Ingredients (for eight servings)

8 eggs
8 thin slices deli-style cooked ham
1 ounce of mozzarella cheese or ¼ cup shredded Italian cheese blend
8 teaspoons basil pesto
8 halved cherry tomatoes or grape tomatoes
Ground black pepper
(Note: you will need muffin cups and nonstick cooking spray)

Preparation
Preheat oven to 350 degrees F.

Coat eight 2 1/2-inch muffin cups with cooking spray. Gently press a ham slice onto the bottom and up the sides of each prepared muffin cup, carefully ruffling the edges of ham.
Divide cheese among the ham-lined muffin cups.

Break an egg into a measuring cup and slip egg into a muffin cup. Repeat with the remaining eggs. Sprinkle with pepper. Spoon 1 teaspoon of the pesto onto each egg (not mandatory). Top with tomato halves.

Bake for 19 minutes or until whites are completely set and yolks are thickened. Let stand in muffin cups for 3 to 5 minutes before serving.

Asparagus and Prosciutto Frittata

Preparation time: 24 minutes

Ingredients (for four servings)
8 eggs
1 cup chopped prosciutto
1/3 cup shredded cheddar cheese (1 to 2 ounces)
½ cup milk
1 tablespoon snipped fresh thyme or 1 teaspoon crushed dried thyme
2 tablespoons olive oil
6 fresh trimmed and cut asparagus spears (cut into 1 1/2-inch pieces)
1/8 teaspoon ground black pepper

Preparation
Preheat broiler. In a medium bowl combine eggs, milk, thyme, and pepper.
Beat with a whisk until well mixed and evenly colored. Set aside.

In a large broiler-proof skillet heat oil over medium heat. Add asparagus;
cook and stir about 4 minutes or until asparagus is crisp-tender. Stir in
prosciutto. Pour egg mixture over asparagus mixture in skillet. Cook over
medium heat. As egg mixture sets, run a spatula around edges of skillet,
lifting egg mixture so the uncooked portion flows underneath.

Continue cooking and lifting edges until egg mixture is almost set (surface
will be moist).
Place skillet under the broiler, 4 to 5 inches from the heat. Broil for up to 2
minutes or just until top is set. Sprinkle with cheese.

Sandwich with feta, spinach and tomato

Preparation time: 18 minutes

Ingredients (for four servings)
4 multigrain sandwich thins
4 eggs
4 tablespoons reduced-fat feta cheese
1 tablespoon snipped fresh rosemary (alternatively 1/2 teaspoon dried rosemary)
2cups fresh baby spinach leaves
1medium tomato, cut into 8 thin slices
1/8 teaspoon salt
4 teaspoons olive oil

Preparation
Preheat oven to 375 degrees F.

Split sandwich thins and brush cut sides with 2 teaspoons of the olive oil. Place on baking sheet and toast in oven 5 minutes or until edges are light brown and crisp. Meanwhile, in a large skillet, heat the remaining 2 teaspoons olive oil and the rosemary over medium-high heat. Break eggs, one at a time, into skillet. Cook 1 minute or until whites are set, but yolks are still runny. Break yolks with spatula. Flip eggs and cook on other side until done. Remove from heat.

Place the bottom halves of the toasted sandwich thins on four serving plates. Divide spinach among sandwich thins on plates. Top each with two of the tomato slices, an egg and 1 tablespoon of the feta cheese. Sprinkle with salt and pepper. Top with the remaining sandwich thin halves.

Raspberry-Java Bulgur

Preparation time: 10 minutes

Ingredients
2/3 cup plain low-fat yogurt (alternative: plain whole-milk Greek yogurt)
¼ cup bulgur
¼ cup raspberries
½ teaspoon instant espresso powder
3 tablespoons milk or refrigerated coconut milk
2 tablespoons packed brown sugar

Preparation
In a bowl stir together all ingredients (except raspberries). Divide mixture between two half-pint jars. Top with raspberries. Cover and chill overnight or up to 3 days. Stir before serving.

Mediterranean Egg Scramble

Preparation time: 30 minutes

Ingredients (for four servings)
6 eggs
4 slices crusty bread
3 thinly sliced medium-sized new potatoes
1/4 large small diced red bell pepper
8 black olives, chopped
1/4 cup chopped fresh parsley
1/4 cup fresh ricotta cheese
1 teaspoon olive oil
1 teaspoon butter
4 teaspoons butter or extra-virgin olive oil
Salt and pepper to taste

Preparation

In a large nonstick skillet, heat the olive oil and butter to medium-high heat. Add the sliced potatoes and sauté until golden (not more than 15 minutes). Add the bell pepper and olives and cook for another 3-4 minutes. In a medium bowl, whisk together eggs, parsley, and ricotta.

Pour the egg mixture over the potato mixture, stirring every 30 seconds until firm and set but not dry (about 3 minutes). Salt and pepper the egg scramble to taste. Serve with crusty bread, lightly toasted and buttered with 1 teaspoon of butter or lightly brushed with 1 teaspoon of extra-virgin olive oil per slice.

Oatmeal with honey roasted plums

Preparation time: 23 minutes

Ingredients (for three servings)
2 cups rolled oats
4 halved and pitted plums
2 tablespoons honey
½ cup chopped roasted pistachios
¼ teaspoon salt

Preparation
Preheat oven to 375F and line a baking sheet with parchment. Place plums face-up up on baking sheet and drizzle with honey. Bake plums no more than 20 minutes, until tender and caramelized. While plums are roasting, cook oatmeal according to package directions. Portion oatmeal into bowls and top with roasted plums. Top with pistachios, and an extra drizzle of honey.

Apple Tahini Toast

Preparation time: 8 minutes

Ingredients (for four servings)
8 slices wholegrain bread
8 tablespoons of tahini
2 thinly sliced apples
1/2 teaspoon cinnamon
2 tablespoons of honey

Preparation
Toast slices of bread to desire doneness. Top east slice with 1.5 tablespoons tahini, half the apple slices, cinnamon and a drizzle of honey.

Avocado and Pumpkin Muffins

Preparation time: 21 minutes

Ingredients (for twelve servings)
2 eggs
1/2 cup mashed avocado
1 1/2 cup pumpkin puree
2 cups flour
1 cup sugar
1 teaspoon baking soda
1 teaspoon salt
1 teaspoon cinnamon
1 teaspoon vanilla extract
1/2 cup of chopped walnuts

Preparation
Preheat oven to 375 F. Grease a muffin tin or line with paper cups. In a large bowl, mix pumpkin, avocado and eggs.

In a separate bowl, whisk sugar, flour, baking soda, salt, cinnamon and vanilla. Combine with avocado mixture, but do not over-mix. Stir in walnuts. Spoon batter into prepared muffin tin and bake for no more than 18 minutes or until tops start to brown and a knife inserted into a muffin comes out clean.

Broccoli Smoothie

Preparation time: 2 minutes

Ingredients (for two servings)
2-3 frozen broccoli florets
1 chopped banana
1 chopped peach
1 cup coconut milk
1 cup cut pineapple
1 teaspoon cinnamon

Preparation
Combine all ingredients in a blender and blend until smooth.

Greek Fluffy Pancakes

Preparation time: 14 minutes

Ingredients (for four servings)
1 egg
½ cup of low-fat yogurt
1 cup buckwheat (or whole-wheat pancake mix)

Preparation
Combine all ingredients until well-mixed. Cook the pancakes following the instructions on the pancake mixture package. Serve pancakes with 2 tablespoons of light maple syrup with a side of 1 of cup fresh strawberries and 1 cup of fat-free milk. Do not eat more than 5 pancakes for one serving.

Breakfast Couscous

Preparation time: 17 minutes

Ingredients (for four servings)
1 cup uncooked whole wheat couscous
3 cups skim milk
¼ cup raisins and currants
½ cup dried apricots
4 teaspoon butter
One cinnamon stick
6 teaspoons brown sugar
Pinch of salt

Preparation
In a pan, combine milk and cinnamon. Boil for 2-3 minutes, stirring continuously. Remove from heat and add couscous, currants, the dried fruits and salt. Add 4 teaspoon of brown sugar to the pan. Mix well. Cover and keep aside for about 15 minutes. Pour into 4 serving bowls. Add teaspoon of butter and ½ tsp brown sugar on top of each bowl before serving.

Italian Tofu Scramble

Preparation time: 23 minutes

Ingredients (for four servings)
1 package of crumbled firm tofu
1-2 teaspoon ground cumin
1 diced zucchini
1 bell diced pepper
1 diced onion
½ cup nutritional yeast
2 teaspoon tamari
2 teaspoon extra-virgin olive oil

Preparation
Mix first tofu, cumin, yeast and tamari with a fork. In a heavy skillet, combine pepper, zucchini, onion and olive oil. Sauté for 5 minutes. Stir in tofu mix and cook for another 10 minutes before serving.

Lunch Recipes

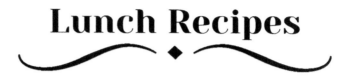

Mediterranean avocado and couscous salad

Preparation time: 27 minutes

Ingredients (for four servings)
1 cup couscous (Israeli or similar)
1 chopped red bell pepper
1 cup cooked black beans
12 oz yellow sweet corn
4 chopped scallions
2 tablespoon of chopped cilantro
Juice of 1 lime
½ cup salsa
Salt and pepper, to taste

Preparation
Cook the couscous according to the package directions and let cool when finished. In a large bowl, combine other ingredients. Season with salt and pepper. Stir in the couscous and mix.

Whole Wheat Fusilli with Kale Pesto

Preparation time: 28 minutes

Ingredients (for four servings)
4 ounces chopped kale
8 ounces whole wheat fusilli
⅓ cup toasted pine nuts
2 ounces grated Parmigiano-Reggiano cheese
2 cloves minced garlic
Salt and pepper, to taste

Preparation
Bring a large pot of salted water to a boil. Add the kale to the boiling water and cook for 5 minutes until it becomes limp. Spread it on a clean cloth. In the same water cook the fusilli according to the instructions. Blend remaining ingredients to make a cream-like mixture. Toss all components and serve.

Tabouli

Preparation time: 29 minutes

Ingredients
1/2 cup fine bulgur wheat
1 de-stemmed bunch of parsley
1 bunch of sliced thinly scallions
1 bunch de-stemmed mint
3 medium diced tomatoes
Juice of 1 lemon
1/3 cup extra virgin olive oil
salt and pepper, to taste

Preparation
After washing, add bulgur to 1 cup of very hot water. Let soak for 20 minutes, while finely chopping herbs. Drain water from bulgur (1st drain and then squeeze in a colander). Add bulgur to chopped vegetables and herbs. Mix in lemon juice and olive oil. Add salt and pepper to taste.

Cretan Pasta with Salmon

Preparation time: 27 minutes

Ingredients (for six servings)
4 salmon steaks (1 ½ - 2 pounds), cut in large cubes
1 pound dry spaghetti
1 shredded medium onion
2 finely chopped cloves garlic
1 cup chopped fresh parsley
1 cup diced tomatoes
1 cup thinly sliced mushrooms
1 teaspoon sweet chili flakes
Salt and pepper, to taste
1/2 cup extra virgin olive oil
Shredded Parmesan cheese, to taste

Preparation
Heat olive oil in deep frying pan. Add onion and sauté for 2 minutes. Add garlic, parsley and a pinch of salt and pepper. Sauté for another minute.

Begin cooking spaghetti according to package directions. Add salmon, tomatoes, mushrooms and chili flakes. Simmer for up to 15 minutes (until salmon is done and mushrooms are tender). Salt and pepper, to taste. Top cooked pasta with vegetables and salmon. Sprinkle with cheese and serve.

Cod with Heirloom Tomato and Plum Sauce

Preparation time: 30 minutes

Ingredients (for four servings)
4 small cod loins
2 cups heirloom tomatoes (chopped in large chunks)
2 tablespoon divided olive oil
8 chopped plums (large chunks)
1 inch piece ginger (pressed)
1 teaspoon Aleppo pepper
1 tablespoon butter
1/4 cup white wine
salt and pepper to taste
chopped parsley (for garnish)

Preparation
Season cod loins with salt and pepper and set aside.

Add 1 tablespoon of olive oil to a frying pan and allow to heat up for 2 minutes. Add tomatoes, plums, ginger and Aleppo pepper. Add salt and pepper to taste. Cook for no more than 15 minutes on medium, stirring occasionally. Add 1 tablespoon of butter and the remaining olive oil to another frying pan. Heat up for two minutes then add the cod loins to the pan. Cook for about 3 minutes on each side until just turning flaky. Add wine to frying pan and cook for an additional two minutes. Serve cod covered with tomato and plum sauce. Garnish with parsley.

Grilled Scallops

Preparation Time: 30 minutes

Ingredients (for four servings)
2 pounds sea scallops
2 tablespoons extra-virgin olive oil
1 tablespoon of melted butter
Zest and juice of 1 lemon
2 tablespoons finely chopped parsley
4 cloves of chopped garlic
Nonstick cooking spray
1/4 teaspoon sea salt

Preparation
Rinse the scallops under water and pat dry. Toss scallops with the garlic, olive oil, butter, and parsley. Allow the scallops to marinate for 10 minutes.

Spray the grill with nonstick cooking spray and heat the grill over medium-high heat. Skewer the scallops and grill them for 1 to 3 minutes on each side or until slightly firm to the touch and opaque. Drizzle with the lemon juice and top with the lemon zest and sea salt just before serving.

Sautéed Broccoli Rabe

Preparation Time: 20 minutes

Ingredients (for six servings)
2 pounds broccoli rabe
1/2 cup chicken stock
4 cloves garlic
1/4 teaspoon red pepper flakes
2 tablespoons extra-virgin olive oil

Preparation
Remove the leaves on the broccoli rabe stem and set them aside. Cut the stalk into 3-inch pieces. In a skillet, heat the olive oil over medium-high heat. Sauté the broccoli rabe stalks and leaves and the garlic for 3 minutes. Add the chicken stock and red pepper flakes and bring to a simmer. Cover and cook for 10 minutes.

Curry-Roasted Cauliflower

Preparation time: 30 minutes

Ingredients (for six servings)
1 head cauliflower
1 tablespoon curry powder
1 tablespoon paprika
1 teaspoon ground coriander
1 teaspoon ground cumin
1/4 cup extra-virgin olive oil
1/2 cup red wine vinegar
1 teaspoon salt

Preparation
Preheat the oven to 425 degrees F.

Cut the cauliflower (including the stalk and leaves) into bite-sized pieces and place in a bowl. In a small bowl, whisk the remaining ingredients. Pour over the cauliflower and toss to coat. Pour the cauliflower and sauce onto a baking sheet and bake for 30 minutes (or more if needed), stirring every 5 minutes.

Grilled Romaine with Lemon Anchovy Dressing

Preparation Time: 10 minutes

Ingredients (for six servings)
4 anchovies, canned in oil
1/2 cup finely chopped fresh parsley
1 large head romaine lettuce, cut in half lengthwise
3 tablespoons freshly grated Parmesan cheese
Juice of 1/2 a medium lemon
1 teaspoon Dijon mustard
2 cloves smashed garlic
1/4 cup plus 1 teaspoon extra-virgin olive oil
Salt to taste

Preparation
Chop the anchovies, lemon juice, parsley, Dijon, and garlic in a small bowl, then put in a blender or food processor for 1 minute. Turn on the machine and slowly drizzle in 1/4 cup of the olive oil until combined, about 2 minutes. Using a piece of the lettuce, taste the dressing and season with salt (if desired).

Heat a grill or grill pan over medium-high heat. Brush the lettuce with the remaining olive oil and grill the cut side for up to 3 minutes, or until grill lines appear.

Roughly chop the grilled lettuce and toss in a large serving bowl with a little dressing at a time until coated. Top with the Parmesan and serve immediately. Save the remaining dressing in the refrigerator and use within 3-4 days.

Mussels with tomatoes and basil

Preparation time: 20 minutes

Ingredients (for six servings)
2 pounds cleaned mussels
One 14.8-ounce can chopped tomatoes
1/4 cup basil, thinly sliced
6 slices crusty French bread
1 tablespoon olive oil
1 chopped onion
2 chopped celery stalks
6 chopped cloves garlic
1/2 teaspoon dried oregano
1 teaspoon red pepper flakes
1 teaspoon honey
2 cups white wine
Salt and pepper to taste

Preparation
In a medium saucepan, heat the olive oil over medium heat.
Add the onions, celery, and garlic and cook for 5 minutes. Add the oregano, tomatoes, crushed red peppers, and honey. Simmer for 10 minutes. Meanwhile, bring the mussels and wine to a boil in a large skillet. Cover and simmer for 10 minutes or until the mussels open. Pour the wine and mussels into the tomato sauce and stir. Season with salt and pepper to taste. Top with the basil and serve with the crusty French bread.

Roasted Black Eyed Beans with Tuna and Pancetta

Preparation time: 28 minutes

Ingredients (for four servings)
1 small jar Italian tuna
1 can black eyed beans
3 tablespoon diced, panfryed pancetta
1 cut in half and then sliced onion
1/2 teaspoon dill
1/4 teaspoon garlic powder
1/2 teaspoon Aleppo pepper
1/4 cup olive oil
salt and pepper to taste

Preparation
Preheat oven to 375 F.

Carefully mix together tuna, garlic powder, the black-eyed beans, onion, Aleppo pepper and dill. Place all of these ingredients in a small oven-proof casserole dish. Cover dish with olive oil, then top with pancetta. Roast for 20 minutes.

Garlicky Curry Chicken Salad

Preparation time: 14 minutes

Ingredients (for four servings)
1 chopped grilled chicken breast
4 large lettuce leaves
2 thinly sliced scallions
1 stalk chopped celery
¼ cup mayonnaise
¼ cup chopped toasted hazelnuts
¼ cup currants
¼ teaspoon curry powder
1/8 teaspoon garlic powder
1/8 teaspoon onion powder
¼ teaspoon aleppo pepper
Salt & Pepper to taste

Preparation
Mix together all ingredients except the lettuce. Serve curried chicken salad atop the lettuce leaves.

Bean Burgers with Garlic and Sage

Preparation time: 20 minutes

Ingredients (for five servings)
One 29 oz. can rinsed and drained pink beans
2 eggs
½ onion minced
1 cup chopped parsley
¾ cup chickpea flour
½ teaspoon black pepper
½ teaspoon dried sage
½ cup olive oil
1 teaspoon salt
1 teaspoon oregano, dried
2 minced garlic cloves

Preparation
In a bowl, mash beans well with a fork, but don't puree. Stop mashing when beans can be easily formed into a ball without falling apart. Add all other ingredients (except olive oil). Blend well with a fork.

Heat oil on medium heat. Form bean mixture into patties. Fry until golden brown on one side and then flip and fry the same on the other side. Drain on paper towels.

Grilled Shrimp Salad with Fresh Dill Dressing

Preparation time: 30 minutes

Ingredients
1 pound shrimp, shelled and de-veined
Juice of 1/2 lemon
2 tablespoons extra virgin olive oil
1/4 teaspoon salt

For dressing:
1/2 cup fresh de-stemmed and chopped dill
1/2 cup extra virgin olive oil
Juice of 1/2 lemon
1/4 teaspoon salt

For salad:
1 yellow pepper, sliced into long strips
1/4 small red onion, sliced in half and then thin rounds
2 Tomatoes, sliced into salad wedges
1 sliced avocado
1 red pepper, sliced into long strips

Preparation
Add the marinade to the shrimp in a bowl or Ziploc bag. Stir or shake well and let the shrimp marinate for at least 30 minutes in the refrigerator. If you have enough time, you can leave it up to 120 minutes.

Prepare the salad dressing by adding the dressing ingredients to a jar and shaking.

Grill the shrimp on a medium-hot grill. Cook on both sides to desired taste, but not more than couple of minutes. Try not to flip the shrimp too many times. Top the salad with grilled shrimp and pour on dressing. Serve immediately.

Grilled Swordfish with Lemon Parsley Topping

Preparation time: 20 minutes

Ingredients (for six servings)
1 1/2 pounds swordfish steaks
1/2 cup chopped parsley
1/2 cup chopped onions
1/2 cup fresh lemon juice
1/2 cup extra virgin olive oil
Salt and pepper, to taste

Preparation
Wash swordfish well and make sure it is dry before putting on grill. Lightly salt.

Mix onions, lemon juice, parsley, salt, olive oil and pepper in a bowl.

Grill swordfish until firm to the touch (anywhere from 3-5 minutes on each side depending on thickness). Cook less if you enjoy your swordfish a bit rarer. Remove from grill and top with lemon parsley mixture.

Cretan Chickpea and Spinach Salad with Avocado

Preparation time: 20 minutes

Ingredients (for six servings)
1 pound of boiled or canned chickpeas
3 chopped tomatoes
1 sliced avocado
1 sliced onion
1 cup sliced mushrooms
1 pound fresh spinach
1 chopped red pepper
1 bunch chopped fresh cilantro
Salt and pepper
1/2 cup of extra virgin olive oil
balsamic vinegar

Preparation
Place the avocado, chickpeas, tomatoes, spinach, onion, mushrooms, red pepper, and cilantro in a bowl. Add salt, pepper, olive oil, and balsamic vinegar to taste. Mix well and serve.

Pan-Fried Scallops with Hand-Chopped Pesto

Preparation time: 25 minutes

Ingredients (for four servings)
1 pound fresh scallops
4 cloves garlic
¼ cup extra virgin olive oil
Salt and pepper, to taste

For the Hand-Chopped Pesto
1 large bunch of basil, washed, de-stemmed and dried with a paper towel.
3 cloves chopped garlic
¼ cup pine nuts or walnuts
⅓ cup shredded parmesan cheese
¼ - ½ cup extra virgin olive oil
Salt, to taste

Preparation
Prepare pesto by placing basil on a large cutting board. Begin chopping the basil with a sharp knife. Add pine nuts, garlic, parmesan cheese and top with about ¼ cup of the olive oil. Keep chopping all of the ingredients until they begin to fold in together. Taste the pesto and decide if you need more of any ingredient. Adding up to another 1/4 cup of olive oil is highly recommended. Continue chopping and add salt.

Heat ¼ cup olive oil on medium heat in a skillet until oil just starts to bubble. Add scallops and a pinch of salt and pepper. Add garlic after about a minute of frying. Fry until scallops begin to brown on the outside and are cooked through on the inside. Add pesto to the pan of scallops. Serve immediately.

Cretan village salad

Preparation time: 5 minutes

Ingredients
2 vine-ripened tomatoes, cut into wedges
2 roughly peeled Lebanese cucumbers, halved lengthways and coarsely chopped
1 thinly sliced Spanish onion
1 cup (loosely packed) purslane or caper leaves or small basil leaves
20 sun-dried black olives
1/2 cup olive oil
Piece of Greek feta
½ teaspoon dried Greek oregano

Preparation
Combine cucumber, tomato, onion, barley rusk, purslane, olives and olive oil in a bowl, season to taste and toss to combine. Arrange on a plate, top with feta, drizzle with extra oil, scatter with Greek oregano and serve.

Avocado Salad with Radish and Cucumber

Preparation time: 15 minutes

Ingredients (for four servings)
2 chopped medium sized radishes
1 large cucumber, cut into quarters lengthwise and then chopped
1/4 cup chopped fresh parsley
1/4 cup chopped red onion
1 ripe avocado, cut into small chunks
Juice of 1/2 lemon
1/2 teaspoon dried dill
3 tablespoons extra virgin olive oil buy now
Salt, to taste

Preparation
Add all ingredients into a large salad bowl. Toss well and serve.

Quinoa Salad with Cucumber and Olives

Preparation time: 30 minutes

Ingredients (for five servings)
1 cup dried quinoa
1 diced English cucumber
1/2 finely chopped red onion
1 can drained and finely chopped black olives
1 cup extra virgin olive oil
1/4 cup red wine vinegar
1 tablespoon lemon juice
2 tablespoons Dijon mustard
2 cups water
Salt and pepper, to taste

Preparation
Wash the quinoa in a strainer. Add the quinoa and water to a saucepot and bring to a boil. As soon as it reaches a boil, turn to low and cook covered for 15 minutes. Let sit for 5 minutes covered after you turn the heat off.

Blend up the Dijon, oil, vinegar and lemon juice in a food processor. If you don't have a food processor, whisk very well until everything is completely emulsified.

In a bowl, mix together the cooked quinoa, diced vegetables, and dressing (to taste). Salt and pepper, to taste. You can serve immediately or let it cool in the fridge during the summer.

Shrimp Salad with Lemon and Parsley

Preparation time: 25 minutes

Ingredients (for six servings)
1 lb. boiled and peeled shrimp
1 sliced thinly head lettuce
3 chopped scallions
1/2 cup chopped parsley, chopped
1/2 cup lemon juice
1/2 cup extra virgin olive oil
salt and pepper

Preparation
In a bowl add lettuce, shrimps and scallions. In a jar add the oil, salt, pepper, parsley and lemon juice. Mix well. Add to bowl with shrimp and toss well.

Prosciutto Wrapped Dates with Sage

Preparation time: 20 minutes

Ingredients (for four servings)
1/3 cup soft goat cheese
2 tablespoon finely chopped fresh sage
10 dates, cut in half
1/8 to 1/4 pound thinly sliced prosciutto (4-6 slices)

Preparation
Combine the cheese and sage in a small bowl and mix well. Generously stuff the cheese mixture into the date halves. Each date half should get about a teaspoon.

Slice the prosciutto into 20 approximately equal pieces and wrap each slice around one of the stuffed date halves.

Heat a skillet over medium heat. Once it's hot, place the prosciutto-wrapped dates in the pan and cook, rotating occasionally, until browned (about 4 minutes). Serve hot.

Grilled Salmon Salad with Yogurt Dill Dressing

Preparation time: 30 minutes

Ingredients (for six servings)
1 1/2 pounds salmon filet

The dressing:
½ cup Greek yogurt
2 tablespoons extra virgin olive oil buy now
2 tablespoons freshly squeezed lemon juice
¼ cup chopped fresh dill
1 tablespoon Dijon mustard
2 teaspoons honey
1/8 teaspoon salt
¼ teaspoon black pepper

The salad:
2 cups mesclun salad mix
1 cucumber, peeled and sliced
2 grated carrots
1/4 of a red onion, sliced into thin rings
2 sliced thin radishes

Preparation
Place salmon on a cookie sheet or large platter. Sprinkle salt and pepper on both sides of the salmon. Let sit while preparing dressing and salad.

Whisk all of the salad dressing ingredients in a bowl.

In a salad bowl or platter that will fit the salmon, add all of the salad vegetables.
Cook the salmon filet skin side up (if there is skin) first on the grill. Grill for about 5 minutes (timing depends on heat and thickness of salmon and desired doneness) on one side and then carefully flip. Grill on the skin side

until done. Remove salmon from grill and top salad with salmon. Drizzle on dressing.

Spinach Fettuccine with Medjool Date Pesto

Preparation time: 30 minutes

Ingredients (for eight servings)
1 pound spinach fettuccine pasta
⅓ cup walnut pieces
3 garlic cloves
½ cup chopped Medjool dates
½ cup crumbled feta cheese
¼ cup extra-virgin olive oil
Salt, to taste

Preparation
Cook pasta according to package directions. Chop the dates, walnuts, and garlic in food processor. While chopping, pour the olive oil. Add cheese and salt to taste. Combine pesto and pasta.

Roasted Vegetable Kebabs

Preparation time: 20 minutes

Ingredients (for eight servings)
cups zucchini
2 cups mushrooms
2 cups onions
2 cups bell peppers
2 tablespoon olive oil
1 tablespoon roasted garlic & herb seasoning

Preparation
Cut vegetables into pieces and toss them with seasoning and oil. Thread the vegetables onto skewers. Grill up to 15 minutes on medium heat until tender.

Stuffed Baked Potato

Preparation time: 30 minutes

Ingredients (for two servings)
2 large Russet potatoes
½ cup non-dairy milk
4 tablespoon oil-free hummus
1 cup chopped cooked vegetables
½ teaspoon hot sauce
Salt, pepper, to taste

Preparation
Preheat oven to 375°F. Bake the potatoes for 1 hour. Split in half and scoop out flesh. Mash the potato flesh with the remaining ingredients. Spoon mixture back into the potato shells. Bake for 15 minutes and serve immediately.

Stuffed Tomatoes with Cheese and Bread Crumbs

Preparation time: 30 minutes

Ingredients (for four servings)
4 medium-large tomatoes
3/4 cup breadcrumbs
1 batch vegan cheddar cheese sauce
1/2 teaspoon onion powder
Salt and pepper, to taste

Preparation
Preheat oven to 350°F. Cut off the top of tomatoes, season with salt and pepper.
Combine the remaining ingredients. Spoon the mixture on the top of each tomato. Bake on baking sheet for 20 minutes and serve.

Salmon and Bean Stir Fry

Preparation time: 10 minutes

Ingredients
1-pound salmon chopped into small cubes
2 cups mung sprouts
1 bunch sliced scallions
2 tablespoon each rice vinegar
2 tablespoon black bean garlic sauce
1 tablespoon dry sherry
2 tablespoon corn flour
1 tablespoon olive oil
¼ cup water

Preparation
In a small bowl, mix vinegar, water, corn flour, bean garlic sauce, and sherry.

In a large skillet, heat the oil and add the salmon cubes. Fry the pieces until browned. Add the mung bean sprouts, scallions and the bean garlic sauce mixture. Stir to coat the salmon pieces. Cook for 2-3 minutes until the sprouts are tender. Serve with sautéed veggies or brown rice.

Vegetable Pita Sandwich with Greek Yogurt Cucumber Sauce

Preparation time: 7 minutes

Ingredients
One-half cup plain light yogurt
1/2 cucumber, finely chopped
1/2 minced garlic clove
1 piece 6 1/2- inch whole-wheat pita
5 halved grape tomatoes
1 cup of string beans
1 cup (22-24 pieces) fresh cherries
Salt & pepper, to taste

Preparation
Mix cucumber, yogurt and garlic until combined, seasoning with salt and pepper, if desired. Spread 1/2 of the sauce on the pita pocket. Fill the pocket with the beans and tomatoes and serve with the cherries.

Tuna Pasta

Preparation time: 5 minutes

Ingrediens
1 cup cooked whole-wheat pasta
3 ounces drained white tuna from can
1 1/2 tablespoons light mayonnaise
Sprinkle of ground black pepper
One-fourth cup chopped bell pepper
One-fourth cup chopped onion
1 fresh plum, to taste

Preparation
Combine all of the ingredients and serve with the plum.

Dinner Recipes

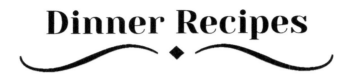

Chicken Kebabs

Preparation time: 30 minutes

Ingredients
4 ounces raw chicken breast, sliced into small-sized chunks
1/4 cup fat-free Italian dressing
1/4 cup white onion
1/4 cup green pepper
10 grape tomatoes
1 piece 6-inch whole-wheat pita
2 tablespoons hummus

Preparation
Put the chicken chunks in a bowl. Add the Italian dressing and toss to coat well. Transfer the bowl in the fridge and let marinate for at least 30 minutes or overnight.

Slice white onion and green pepper and into chunks. Wash and clean the cherry tomatoes.
Alternate the green pepper, cherry tomatoes, white onion, and marinated chicken on skewers and grill until the chicken is cooked.

When the kebabs are grilled, grill the pita until toasted. Brush the toasted pita with 2 tablespoons hummus. Serve the kebab with the pita.

Walnut-Rosemary Crusted Salmon

Preparation time: 30 minutes

Ingredients (for four servings)
2 teaspoons Dijon mustard
1 minced clove garlic
¼ teaspoon lemon zest
1 teaspoon lemon juice
1 teaspoon chopped fresh rosemary
½ teaspoon honey
½ teaspoon salt
¼ teaspoon crushed red pepper
3 tablespoons panko breadcrumbs
3 tablespoons finely chopped walnuts
1 teaspoon extra-virgin olive oil
1 (1 pound) fresh or frozen skinless salmon fillet
Olive oil cooking spray

Preparation
Preheat oven to 425°F.

Line a large rimmed baking sheet with parchment paper. Combine garlic, mustard, lemon juice, lemon zest, honey, rosemary, salt. and crushed red pepper in a small bowl.

Combine oil, panko. and walnuts in another small bowl. Place salmon on the prepared baking sheet. Spread the mustard mixture over the fish and sprinkle with the panko mixture, pressing to adhere. Lightly coat with cooking spray. Bake until the fish flakes easily with a fork, about 9 to 13 minutes, depending on thickness.

Greek Salad Nachos

Preparation time: 14 minutes

Ingredients (for six servings)
⅓ cup prepared hummus
2 tablespoons extra-virgin olive oil
1 tablespoon lemon juice
¼ teaspoon ground pepper
3 cups whole-grain pita chips
1 cup chopped romaine lettuce
½ cup quartered grape tomatoes
¼ cup crumbled feta cheese
2 tablespoons chopped Kalamata olives
2 tablespoons minced red onion
1 tablespoon minced fresh oregano

Preparation
Whisk hummus, oil, lemon juice and pepper in a small bowl. Spread pita chips in one layer on a platter. Drizzle ¾ of the hummus mixture over the chips. Top with lettuce, feta, tomatoes, red onion and olives. Dollop with the remaining hummus mixture and sprinkle with oregano.

Chicken with Tomato-Balsamic Pan Sauce

Preparation time: 30 minutes

Ingredients (for four servings):
2 8-ounce boneless and skinless chicken breasts
1 cup low-sodium chicken broth
½ teaspoon ground pepper
¼ cup white whole-wheat flour
½ cup halved cherry tomatoes
2 tablespoons sliced shallot
¼ cup balsamic vinegar
1 tablespoon minced garlic
1 tablespoon fennel seeds
3 tablespoons extra-virgin olive oil
½ teaspoon salt
toasted and lightly crushed 1 tablespoon butter

Preparation
Remove and reserve chicken tenders (if any) for another use. Slice each breast in half horizontally to make 4 pieces total. Place on a cutting board and cover with a large piece of plastic wrap. Pound with the smooth side of a meat mallet or a heavy saucepan to an even thickness of about ¼ inch. Sprinkle with ¼ teaspoon each salt and pepper.

Place flour in a shallow dish and dredge the cutlets to coat both sides, shaking off excess. (Discard remaining flour.)

Heat 2 tablespoons oil in a large skillet over medium-high heat. Add 2 pieces of chicken and cook, turning once, until evenly browned and cooked through, up to 3 minutes per side. Transfer to a large serving plate and tent with foil to keep warm. Repeat with the remaining chicken.

Add the remaining 1 tablespoon oil, tomatoes and shallot to the pan. Cook, stirring occasionally, until softened, 1 to 2 minutes. Add vinegar and bring to a boil. Cook, scraping up any browned bits from the bottom of the pan, until the vinegar is reduced by about half, about 45 seconds. Add broth, garlic, fennel seeds, and the remaining ¼ teaspoon salt and pepper.

Cook, stirring, until the sauce is reduced by about half, 5 to 7 minutes. Remove from heats and stir in butter. Serve the sauce over the chicken.

Grilled Salmon with Vegetables

Preparation time: 23 minutes

Ingredients (for four servings)
1¼ pounds salmon fillet, cut into 4 portions
1 medium halved lengthwise zucchini
2 trimmed, halved and seeded bell peppers (yellow/orange/red)
1 medium red onion, cut into 1-inch wedges
½ teaspoon salt
½ teaspoon ground pepper
¼ cup thinly sliced fresh basil
1 tablespoon extra-virgin olive oil
1 lemon, cut into 4 wedges

Preparation
Preheat grill to medium-high. Brush zucchini, peppers and onion with oil and sprinkle with ¼ teaspoon salt. Sprinkle salmon with pepper and the remaining ¼ teaspoon salt.

Place the vegetables and the salmon pieces, skin-side down, on the grill. Cook the vegetables, turning once or twice, until just tender and grill marks appear, about 5 minutes per side. Cook the salmon, without turning, until it flakes when tested with a fork, 8 to 10 minutes. When cool enough to handle, roughly chop the vegetables and toss together in a large bowl.

Remove the skin from the salmon fillets (if desired) and serve alongside the vegetables. Garnish each serving with 1 tablespoon basil and serve with a lemon wedge.

Turkey Burger with Tzatziki, Feta and Spinach

Preparation time: 30 minutes

Ingredients (for four servings)
1 cup thawed frozen chopped spinach
4 small whole-wheat hamburger buns
1 pound 93% lean ground turkey
½ cup crumbled feta cheese
4 tablespoons tzatziki
12 slices cucumber
½ teaspoon garlic powder
½ teaspoon dried oregano
¼ teaspoon salt
¼ teaspoon ground pepper

Preparation
Preheat grill to medium-high.

Squeeze excess moisture from spinach. Combine the spinach with feta, turkey, oregano, garlic powder, salt and pepper in a medium bowl. Mix well.

Form into four 4-inch patties. Oil the grill rack by oiling a folded paper towel and hold it with tongs and rub it over the rack.

Grill the patties until cooked through and no longer pink in the center, 4 to 6 minutes per side. (An instant-read thermometer inserted in the center should be 165°F.)

Assemble the burgers on the buns, topping each with 1 tablespoon tzatziki, 2 onion rings and 3 cucumber slices.

Chicken and Spinach Soup with Fresh Pesto

Preparation time: 30 minutes

Ingredients (for five servings)
½ cup carrot or diced red bell pepper
1 large boneless, skinless chicken breast, cut into quarters
5 cups reduced-sodium chicken broth
1 15-ounce can cannellini beans or great northern beans, rinsed
1 large minced clove garlic
1½ teaspoons dried marjoram
6 ounces baby spinach, coarsely chopped
¼ cup grated Parmesan cheese
1 tablespoon and 2 teaspoons extra-virgin olive oil, divided
⅓ cup lightly packed fresh basil leaves
Freshly ground pepper to taste
¾ cup plain or herbed multigrain croutons for garnish (optional)

Preparation

Heat 2 teaspoons oil in a large saucepan or Dutch oven over medium-high heat. Add carrot or bell pepper and chicken. Cook about 4 minutes, turning the chicken and stirring frequently, until the chicken begins to brown.

Add garlic and cook, stirring, for 1 minute more. Stir in broth and marjoram, bring to a boil over high heat. Reduce the heat and simmer, stirring occasionally, until the chicken is cooked through, about 5 minutes.

With a slotted spoon, transfer the chicken pieces to a clean cutting board to cool. Add spinach and beans to the pot and bring to a gentle boil. Cook for 5 minutes to blend the flavors.
Combine the remaining 1 tablespoon oil, Parmesan and basil in a food processor (a mini processor works well). Process until a coarse paste forms, adding a little water and scraping down the sides as necessary.

Cut the chicken into bite-size pieces. Stir the chicken and pesto into the pot. Season with pepper. Heat until hot. Garnish with croutons, if desired.

Mediterranean Edamame Toss

Preparation time: 30 minutes

Ingredients (for four servings)
½ cup rinsed and drained uncooked quinoa
1 cup ready-to-eat fresh or frozen, thawed shelled sweet soybeans (edamame)
¼ cup crumbled reduced-fat feta cheese
2 medium seeded and chopped tomatoes
1 cup fresh arugula or spinach leaves
½ cup chopped red onion
1 teaspoon finely shredded lemon peel
2 tablespoons lemon juice
2 tablespoons snipped fresh basil
¼ teaspoon salt
¼ teaspoon freshly ground black pepper
2 tablespoons olive oil
1 cup water

Preparation
In a medium saucepan, combine quinoa and water. Bring to boiling and then reduce heat. Cover and simmer about 15 minutes or until quinoa is tender and liquid is absorbed, adding edamame the last 4 minutes of cooking.

In a large bowl, combine tomato, quinoa mixture, arugula, and onion. In a small bowl, whisk together olive oil, lemon peel, and lemon juice. Stir in half of the cheese, the basil, salt, and pepper.

Add mixture to quinoa mixture, tossing to coat. Sprinkle with remaining half of the cheese before serving.

Shrimp Piccata with Zucchini Noodles

Preparation time: 30 minutes

Ingredients (for four servings)
1 pound raw peeled and deveined shrimp (21-25 count)
5-6 medium trimmed zucchini (2¼-2½ pounds)
3 tablespoons rinsed capers
2 tablespoons chopped fresh parsley
2 tablespoons extra-virgin olive oil
2 cloves minced garlic
1 cup low-sodium chicken broth
1 tablespoon cornstarch
⅓ cup white wine
¼ cup lemon juice
2 tablespoons butter
½ teaspoon salt

Preparation
Using a spiral vegetable slicer or a vegetable peeler, cut zucchini lengthwise into long, thin strands or strips. Stop when you reach the seeds in the middle (seeds make the noodles fall apart). Place the zucchini "noodles" in a colander and toss with salt. Let drain for 15 to 30 minutes, then gently squeeze to remove any excess water.

Meanwhile, heat butter and 1 tablespoon oil in a large skillet over medium-high heat. Add garlic and cook, stirring, for 30 seconds. Add shrimp and cook, stirring, for 1 minute. Whisk broth and cornstarch in a small bowl. Add to the shrimp along with wine, lemon juice and capers. Simmer, stirring occasionally, until the shrimp is just cooked through, 4 to 5 minutes. Remove from heat.

Heat the remaining 1 tablespoon oil in a large nonstick skillet over medium-high heat. Add the zucchini noodles and gently toss until hot, about 3 minutes. Serve the shrimp and sauce over the zucchini noodles, sprinkled with parsley.

Turkey meatball gyro

Preparation time: 25 minutes

Ingredients (for four servings)
1 lb. ground turkey
1/4 cup finely diced red onion
2 minced garlic cloves
1 teaspoon oregano
1 cup chopped fresh spinach
2 tablespoons olive oil

Tzatziki Sauce
1/2 cup plain Greek yogurt
1/4 cup grated cucumber
1 cup diced tomato
1 cup diced cucumber
4 whole wheat flatbreads
2 tablespoons lemon juice
1/2 teaspoon dry dill
1/2 teaspoon garlic powder
1/2 cup thinly sliced red onion
salt to taste

Instructions
To a large bowl add ground turkey, minced garlic, diced red onion, salt, oregano, fresh spinach and pepper. Using your hands, mix all the ingredients together until meat forms a ball and sticks together. Form meat mixture into 1" balls. In total, you will make 11-13 meatballs.

Heat a large skillet to medium-high heat. Add olive oil to the pan, and then add the meatballs. Cook each side for 3-4 minutes until they are browned on all sides. Remove from the pan and let rest.

In the meantime, to a small bowl add Greek yogurt, dill, grated cucumber, lemon juice, garlic powder and salt to taste. Mix together until everything is combined.

Assemble the gyros: to a flatbread add 3 meatballs, sliced red onion, tomato, and cucumber. Then top with Tzatziki sauce to taste.

Couscous with Tuna and Pepperoncini

Preparation time: 14 minutes

Ingredients (for four servings)
1¼ cups couscous
1 cup chicken broth or water
¾ teaspoon salt

Accompaniments
Two 5-ounce cans oil packed tuna
1 pint halved cherry tomatoes
½ cup sliced pepperoncini
⅓ cup chopped fresh parsley
¼ cup capers
Extra-virgin olive oil
Salt and paper, to taste
1 quartered lemon

Preparation
In a small pot, bring the broth or water to a boil over medium heat. Remove the pot from the heat, stir in the couscous and cover the pot. Let sit for 10 minutes.

Meanwhile, in a medium bowl, toss together pepperoncini, the tuna, tomatoes, parsley and capers.

Fluff the couscous with a fork, season with salt and pepper, and drizzle with olive oil. Top the couscous with the tuna mixture and serve with lemon wedges.

Classic Mediterranean Cod

Preparation time: 30 minutes

Ingredients (for four servings)
2 tablespoon olive oil
1 small sliced onion
2 cups sliced fennel
3 large chopped cloves garlic
1 14.5 ounce can diced tomato
1 cup diced fresh tomatoes
2 cups shredded kale
1/2 cup water
pinch of crushed red pepper
2 teaspoon fresh oregano (or 1/2 teaspoon of dried oregano)
1 cup oil cured black olives
1 lb. cod cut into 4 portions
1/8 teaspoon salt
1/4 teaspoon black pepper
1/4 teaspoon fennel seeds optional
1 teaspoon orange zest
fresh oregano fennel fronds, orange zest, olive oil

Preparation

In a large skillet over medium heat, cook garlic, onion and fennel in olive oil for 8 minutes, season with salt and pepper (about 1/4 teaspoon of each). Add fresh and canned diced tomato, kale, and water. Stir well and cook for 12 minutes. Add crushed red pepper, fresh oregano, and olives.

Prepare fish, season with salt, pepper, orange zest, and fennel seeds. Nestle fish into kale tomato stewing mixture. Cover pan and cook for 10 minutes. Remove from heat, and finish with fennel fronds, more fresh oregano, more orange zest, and a drizzle of olive oil on top and serve.

Smoky Tempeh Tostadas with Mango

Preparation time: 23 minutes

Ingredients (for three servings)
1 8-ounce package tempeh, cut into thin chunks
1/4 cup soy sauce (or liquid aminos)
1 1/2 cups shredded red cabbage
3/4 cup diced mango
1/2 cup cilantro, finely minced, plus more for topping
6 corn tortillas
1 teaspoon chili powder
1/2-1 teaspoon hot sauce
1/2 teaspoon ground cumin
1/2 teaspoon liquid smoke
1/2 teaspoon garlic powder
1/2 teaspoon onion powder
1/4 teaspoon black pepper
1 tablespoon fresh lime juice
1 teaspoon apple cider vinegar
1 teaspoon agave nectar
1/4 teaspoon salt
Oil for cooking

Additional toppings to taste: cilantro, avocado, salsa, lettuce

Preparation
Preheat oven to 350°F. Place the tempeh chunks in a medium bowl.

In a small bowl, add soy sauce, hot sauce, chili powder, onion powder, cumin, liquid smoke, garlic powder, and pepper. Whisk to combine. Pour over tempeh; stir until evenly coated. Set aside for 5-10 minutes.

Place corn tortillas on a baking sheet. Lightly brush with oil. Bake for 10 minutes, until crispy and golden.

In a skillet over medium heat, add the tempeh. Let it cook on side for 4-5 minutes, until browned. Flip the chunks and cook for another 3-4 minutes.

While the tempeh and tortillas are cooking, add red cabbage, agave, mango, cilantro, lime juice, vinegar, and salt to a medium bowl. Stir to combine.

Scoop the tempeh onto the tortillas, then top with slaw and any other desired toppings.

Chickpea and Vegetable Coconut Curry

Preparation time: 28 minutes

Ingredients (for four servings)
¼ cup chopped fresh cilantro
4 scallions, thinly sliced
One 14-ounce can coconut milk
1 red onion, thinly sliced
1 red bell pepper, thinly sliced
One 28-ounce can cooked chickpeas
1½ cups frozen peas
1 tablespoon minced fresh ginger
3 minced garlic cloves
1 small head cauliflower, cut into bite-size florets
2 teaspoons Chile powder
1 teaspoon ground coriander
3 tablespoons red curry paste
1 tablespoon extra-virgin olive oil
1 halved lime
Salt and freshly ground black pepper

Preparation
In a large pot, heat the olive oil over medium heat. Add the onion and bell pepper, and sauté until nearly tender, no more than 5 minutes. Add the ginger and garlic, and sauté until fragrant, about 1 minute.

Add the toss and cauliflower well to combine. Stir in the Chile powder, coriander and red curry paste, and cook until the whole mixture darkens slightly, about 1 minute. Stir in the coconut milk and bring the mixture to a simmer over medium-low heat. Cover the pot and continue to simmer until the cauliflower is tender, 8 to 10 minutes.

Remove the lid and squeeze lime juice into the curry, stirring well to combine. Add the chickpeas and peas, season with salt and pepper, and bring the mixture back to a simmer. Serve with rice, if desired. Garnish each portion with 1 tablespoon cilantro and 1 tablespoon scallions.

Potato Noodles with Almond Sauce

Preparation time: 20 minutes

Ingredients (for four servings)
3 minced shallots
2 minced garlic cloves
3 tablespoons all-purpose flour
2 cups plain, unsweetened almond milk
2 tablespoons Dijon mustard
4 tablespoons extra-virgin olive oil
3 sweet potatoes, cut into noodles
4 cups roughly torn kale
Salt and freshly ground black pepper
½ cup toasted, salted almonds, roughly chopped

Preparation
In a medium pot, heat the 2 tablespoons of olive oil over medium heat. Add the garlic and shallots, and sauté until fragrant, about 1 minute.

Stir in the flour and cook, stirring constantly, for 1 minute. Add the almond milk, whisking constantly to prevent lumps from forming in the sauce. Whisk over medium heat until the mixture comes to a simmer. Simmer for up to 5 minutes.

Whisk in the Dijon mustard and season the sauce with salt and pepper. Cover and continue to warm the sauce over low heat while you prepare the noodles.

In a large sauté pan, heat 2 tablespoon of olive oil over medium heat. Add the sweet potato noodles and sauté, tossing occasionally, until they are nearly tender, 5 to 6 minutes. Add the kale and toss until it wilts. Add the sauce and toss until the noodles are well coated. Before serving, add the almonds and toss to combine and add salt and pepper, to taste.

Mediterranean Kale Quinoa Salad

Preparation time: 27 minutes

Ingredients (for four servings)
1 cup quinoa
1 cup stems removed baby kale
3 tablespoons Kalamata olives
1 cup quartered cherry tomatoes
1 tablespoon chopped fresh parsley
½ cup diced cucumber
¼ cup minced red onion
2 tablespoons extra virgin olive oil
2 tablespoons lemon juice
⅛ teaspoon salt
⅛ teaspoon pepper
feta cheese to taste
2 cups water

Preparation
Put quinoa to a medium saucepan and add water. Bring to a boil and reduce the heat to a simmer. Cook until all of the liquid is absorbed, 14-15 minutes.

Meanwhile add the rest of the ingredients to a bowl and then toss in cooked quinoa. Serve with a sprinkle of feta cheese.

Spanish Salmon Tacos

Preparation time: 23 minutes

Ingredients (for three servings)
9 corn tortillas
1 (½ pound) piece fresh salmon
1 teaspoon olive oil
Garlic powder, ground cumin, chili powder, salt, paper to taste
1 cup plain Greek yogurt
Juice from 1/2 lime
1 minced clove garlic
Handful fresh chopped cilantro
1 avocado diced
Iceberg lettuce shredded

Preparation
Preheat oven to 375F. Move the rack to the middle position. Line a baking sheet with foil. Wrap the tortillas in foil and put them in the oven right away.

Place a piece of salmon on the baking sheet and coat it with olive oil. Gently sprinkle with garlic powder, ground cumin, chili powder, and salt & pepper, to taste. Cook in oven for 11-14 minutes or until it flakes easily with a fork.

Meanwhile, prepare sauce by combining Greek yogurt, juice from lime, minced garlic and cilantro. Set aside. Prepare the avocado and lettuce.

When the salmon is done, roughly cut it into bite-size pieces using a fork. Assemble tacos immediately. Serve with extra lime to taste.

Lebanese Lemon Chicken

Preparation time: 25 minutes

Ingredients (for seven servings)
3 pounds boneless, skinless chicken thighs (10-14 thighs)
1/2 teaspoon ground turmeric
Freshly ground black pepper
1 large onion
2 sprigs of fresh rosemary
3 lemons
2 tablespoons extra virgin olive oil
1½ teaspoons flaky sea salt
2 sprigs of fresh thyme

Preparation
Juice one of the lemons until you have 2 tablespoons of lemon juice. Put the juice in a bowl and add the 2 tablespoons of olive oil along with the turmeric, sea salt, and a generous amount of freshly ground black pepper.

Add the chicken thighs to the bowl and toss to coat. Let the chicken marinate several minutes at room temperature while you prepare the other ingredients.

Trim the ends off the other two lemons and slice them into ¼-inch thick rounds. Remove any visible seeds. Halve, peel, and slice the onion.

Heat two large cast iron skillets over medium-high heat (or use one skillet and cook the chicken in two batches). Add enough olive oil to coat the bottom with a thin layer of oil. Divide the chicken pieces between the two pans with the smooth side of the chicken (where the skin was) facing down, making sure to leave a little room between the pieces so they can brown. Cook for about 5 minutes, until nicely browned on the bottom, and then flip and cook for about 9 minutes on the second side, until just cooked through, lowering the heat slightly if necessary. Use tongs or a slotted spatula to transfer the chicken pieces to a plate.

Add the lemons, onions, and herb sprigs to the pans. Let cook undisturbed for 3-4 minutes, until the lemons are browned on the bottom. Pour ½ cup water into each pan and stir, scraping the browned bits from the bottom.

Reduce the heat to medium, add the chicken back to the pans, and cook for 4-5 minutes so the flavors can meld. Serve the chicken with onion and pan juices hot over rice.

Creamy chicken

Preparation time: 23 minutes

Ingredients (for five servings)
1½ pounds chicken breasts (about ½ inch thick)
¼ cup julienne cut sun dried tomatoes
1¼ cups half-and-half cream
1 (14 ounce) can drained marinated artichoke hearts
⅓ cup pitted Kalamata olives
¼ cup Parmesan cheese
2 tablespoons sliced fresh basil
2 tablespoons oil
1 teaspoon minced garlic
¼ cup feta cheese

Preparation
Heat oil in a large skillet over medium heat.

Season chicken with salt and pepper and then place in the pan. Cook for no more than 5 minutes until browned and then flip. Cook another 3-4 minutes or until internal temperature is 165 F. Remove chicken from skillet.

Add garlic to skillet and cook for 30 seconds, stirring constantly. Add the olives, cream, artichoke and sun-dried tomatoes.

Bring to a low boil and cook while stirring until slightly thickened. Stir in the Parmesan cheese and then add the chicken back to the pan. Turn off the heat and serve with pasta or rice, garnished with basil and feta.

Italian cobb salad

Preparation time: 9 minutes

Ingredients (for two servings)
4 cups Romaine lettuce
2 thinly sliced hard boiled eggs
2 cups artichoke hearts
1 cup drained marinated roasted red peppers
3/4 cup diced English cucumbers
3/4 cup crumbled feta cheese
1/2 cup Kalamata olives
2 tablespoons fresh basil

Vinaigrette
3 to 4 tablespoons olive oil
1 to 2 tablespoons red wine vinegar
1 tablespoon honey, or to taste
1/2 teaspoon dried oregano
1/2 teaspoon dried basil
1/2 teaspoon dried dill
Salt and pepper, or to taste

Preparation
To a large serving platter, evenly scatter the Romaine, evenly lay down the remaining ingredients in long rows, and evenly sprinkle with fresh basil.

For vinaigrette take a glass jar or container with a lid, add all ingredients, shake vigorously to combine, taste vinaigrette and make any necessary flavor adjustments, then evenly drizzle over salad and serve immediately. Dressing will keep airtight in the fridge for up to 5 days.

Seared Fish with Zucchini Farro

Preparation time: 30 minutes

Ingredients (for two servings)
10½ oz of your favorite mild white fish
½ cup semi-pearled farro
4 oz halved grape or cherry tomatoes
1 oz pitted roughly chopped olives
1 chopped zucchini
2 cloves minced garlic
½ teaspoon oregano
2 tablespoon red wine vinegar
2 tablespoon extra-virgin olive oil
¼ teaspoon crushed red pepper flakes
¼ cup rice
Salt and pepper, to taste

Preparation
Heat a medium pot of salted water to boiling on high. Once boiling, add the farro and cook, uncovered, no more than 20 minutes, or until tender. Drain thoroughly and return to the pot. Meanwhile, combine olives and tomatoes in a medium bowl. Add 1 tablespoon of vinegar and a drizzle of olive oil. Season with salt and pepper and stir to combine.

Pat fish dry with paper towels. Transfer to cutting board and halve each fillet crosswise. Season with salt and pepper on both sides.

In a large pan, heat 2 teaspoon olive oil on medium-high until hot. Add the sliced zucchini in an even layer. Cook, without stirring, 3 to 4 minutes, or until lightly browned. Add the garlic, oregano, and a pinch of red pepper flakes. Season with salt and pepper. Cook, stirring often, until zucchini is softened. Add remaining 1 tablespoon vinegar and cook until liquid has cooked off. Transfer to pot with farro and add a drizzle of olive oil, salt and pepper to taste. Wipe down pan and heat a drizzle of olive oil on medium-high until hot. Meanwhile, place flour on a large plate and season with salt and pepper. Coat the fish in flour. Tap off excess flour and add coated fish to pan. Cook 3-4 minutes per side, or until golden and cooked through. Turn off the heat. Serve farro topped with cooked fish and tomato topping.

Croatian Sheet Pan Salmon

Preparation time: 27 minutes

Ingredients (for six servings)

2-3 pounds whole salmon filet
2 thinly sliced lemons
1/2 cup pitted assorted olives
2 cups halved cherry tomatoes
Marinated sweet or hot peppers
2 teaspoon capers
2 tablespoon salted butter
1/4 thinly sliced red onion
4 tablespoon extra-virgin olive oil
Salt and pepper
Oregano, rosemary, thyme to taste

Preparation
Preheat oven to 425F.

Line baking sheet with parchment paper and lay out your fish. Tuck the thin tail end under to make a thicker layer so the fish will cook evenly. Arrange the lemon slices on and around the fish, along with the onions, olives, peppers, tomatoes and capers. Drizzle olive oil over all, and sprinkle with salt and pepper. Dot with chunks of butter, if using.

Bake for about 25 minutes, or until the fish is done through and flakes easily with a fork. The exact cooking time will depend on the size and thickness of fish, and if your fish is especially thick, or heavier, it will take longer. Garnish with herbs before serving.

Shrimp and Zucchini Fritters

Preparation time: 28 minutes

Ingredients (for four servings)
1/2 lb. peeled and deveined shrimp, roughly chopped
3 grated medium zucchini
1 cup whole wheat Panko breadcrumbs
2 eggs
Zest of one lemon
2 tablespoons minced fresh parsley
2 tablespoons olive oil
Salt and pepper, to taste

Sauce
3/4 cup Greek yogurt
1 large minced clove garlic
Juice of one lemon
1/4 teaspoon salt
1/4 teaspoon pepper

Preparation
Mix together all ingredients for yogurt sauce. Set aside.

Using a clean kitchen towel, squeeze out as much liquid from the grated zucchini as possible. Combine shrimp, zucchini, eggs, breadcrumbs, salt, parsley, pepper, lemon zest, and parsley in a large bowl. Mixture should hold together well—if it seems too wet, add some more breadcrumbs.

Heat the oil in a cast iron or other heavy skillet over medium-high heat. Using a large scoop or a 1/2 cup measure, scoop mixture into hot oil. Flatten tops slightly with a spatula.

Cook for 3 minutes, flip, and cook for another 3 minutes, or until golden brown on both sides. Remove and place on a paper towel lined plate.

Continue until all of zucchini mixture is used up, adding more oil if necessary. Serve fritters with yogurt sauce and lemon wedges.

Quesadillas with Garlic Hummus

Preparation time: 13 minutes

Ingredients
2 flour tortillas
Roasted garlic hummus
Crumbled Feta cheese
Shredded mozzarella cheese
Chopped Kalamata olives
Sliced roasted red peppers
1 teaspoon olive oil
Arugula
Chopped fresh parsley or basil, sliced cherry tomatoes, yogurt, or tzatziki

Preparation
Heat olive oil in a skillet on medium-high heat. Add one tortilla. Sprinkle the top with both cheeses, olives, and roasted red peppers. Cook until cheese is melted.

While the cheesy tortilla is cooking, spread the other tortilla with a layer of hummus. When the cheese is melted, top with handful of arugula followed by the other hummus-smothered tortilla. Using a spatula, carefully flip and cook up to 2 minutes on the other side until slightly crispy. Remove from skillet, cut into wedges and serve.

Pork Marsala

Preparation time: 28 minutes

Ingredients (for six servings)
1/3 cup whole wheat flour
6 boneless pork loin chops
2 chopped turkey bacon strips
1/4 teaspoon minced garlic
1 tablespoon olive oil
2 cups sliced fresh mushrooms
1/3 cup chopped onion
1 cup Marsala wine
1/2 teaspoon pepper
5 teaspoons cornstarch
2/3 cup reduced-sodium chicken broth

Preparation
In a shallow bowl, mix flour and pepper. Dip pork chops in flour mixture to coat both sides and shake off excess.

In a large non-stick skillet coated with cooking spray, heat oil over medium heat. Add pork chops and cook 4-5 minutes on each side or until a thermometer reads 145°. Remove from pan but keep warm.

In same skillet, add onion, mushrooms, and bacon to drippings. Cook and stir 2-3 minutes or until mushrooms are tender. Add garlic and cook 1 minute longer. Add wine and increase heat to medium-high. Cook, stirring to loosen browned bits from pan.

In a small bowl, mix cornstarch and broth until smooth and add to pan. Bring to a boil and cook and stir 2 minutes or until slightly thickened. Serve with pork.

Turkey Skillet

Preparation time: 27 minutes

Ingredients (for six servings)
20 ounces lean ground turkey
2 medium zucchini (quartered lengthwise and cut into 1/2-inch slices)
1 chopped medium onion
2 seeded and chopped peppers
3 minced garlic cloves
1/2 teaspoon dried oregano
15 ounces rinsed and drained black beans
15 ounces undrained diced tomatoes,
1 tablespoon balsamic vinegar
1 tablespoon olive oil
1/2 teaspoon salt

Preparation
In a large skillet, heat oil over medium-high heat. Add onion, peppers and garlic. Add turkey, zucchini and oregano and cook 10-12 minutes, or until turkey is no longer pink and vegetables are tender breaking up turkey into crumbles. Stir in remaining ingredients and heat through, stirring occasionally.

Italian Tilapia

Preparation time: 30 minutes

Ingredients (for four servings)
4 tilapia fillets (6 ounces each)
1/4 teaspoon pepper
15 ounces diced tomatoes with basil, oregano, and garlic
1 large halved and thinly sliced onion
1 medium julienned green pepper
1/4 cup shredded Parmesan cheese

Preparation
Preheat oven to 350°. Place tilapia in a 13x9-inch baking dish coated with cooking spray and sprinkle with pepper. Spoon tomatoes over tilapia and top with onion and green pepper.
Cover and bake 30 minutes. Uncover and sprinkle with cheese. Bake 10 minutes longer or until fish flakes easily with a fork.

Tuna Wraps

Preparation time: 18 minutes

Ingredients (for four servings)
12 ounces light tuna in water (drained and flaked)
15 ounces rinsed and drained cannellini beans
12 Bibb or Boston lettuce leaves
1 peeled and sliced ripe avocado
1/4 cup chopped red onion
2 tablespoons olive oil
1 tablespoon minced fresh parsley
1/8 teaspoon salt
1/8 teaspoon pepper

Preparation
In a bowl, combine all ingredients, except lettuce leaves and avocado and toss lightly to combine. Serve in lettuce leaves; top with avocado.

Fish and Veggie Skillet

Preparation time: 28 minutes

Ingredients (for four servings)
4 fillets (6 ounces each) of fish (tilapia, mahi mahi or salmon)
3 medium sweet red peppers, cut into thick strips
1/2 pound sliced baby Portobello mushrooms
1 large sweet onion, cut into thick rings and separated
1/3 cup lemon juice
3/4 teaspoon salt
1/2 teaspoon pepper
1/4 cup minced fresh chives
3 tablespoons olive oil
1/3 cup pine nuts

Preparation
In a large skillet, heat 2 tablespoons oil over medium-high heat. Add fillets and cook up to 5 minutes on each side or until fish just begins to flake easily with a fork. Remove from pan. Add remaining onion, oil, mushrooms, peppers, lemon juice and 1/4 teaspoon salt. Cook, covered, over medium heat until vegetables are tender, stirring occasionally, 6-8 minutes. Place fish over vegetables and sprinkle with pepper and remaining salt. Cook, covered, 2 minutes longer or until heated through. Sprinkle with chives and pine nuts before serving.

Mediterranean Fish Bake

Preparation time: 30 minutes

Ingredients (for four servings)
4 cod fillets (6 ounces each)
2 tablespoons olive oil
1/4 teaspoon salt
1/8 teaspoon pepper
1 small green pepper, cut into thin strips
1/2 small thinly sliced red onion,
1/4 cup pitted sliced Greek olives
8 ounces tomato sauce
1/4 cup crumbled feta cheese

Preparation
Preheat oven to 400°.
Place cod in a greased 13x9-inch baking dish. Brush with oil and sprinkle with salt and pepper. Top with green pepper, onion, and olives. Pour tomato sauce over top and sprinkle with cheese. Bake until fish just begins to flake easily with a fork, 15-20 minutes.

Snack Recipes

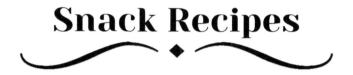

Salmon and Goat Cheese Bits

Preparation time: 5 minutes

Ingredients
1 package smoked salmon
3 endive heads
1 package herbed goat cheese

Preparation
Cut the ends off the endives and pull the leaves apart. Spread goat cheese on endive leaves. Place salmon slices on top of goat cheese.

Banana and Peanut Yogurt

Preparation time: 5 minutes

Ingredients (for four servings)
4 cups vanilla Greek yogurt
1/4 cup creamy natural peanut butter
2 medium bananas sliced
1/4 cup flax seed meal
1 teaspoon nutmeg

Instructions
Divide yogurt between four bowls and top with banana slices. Melt peanut butter in a microwave safe bowl for 30-40 seconds and drizzle one tablespoon on each bowl on top of the bananas. Sprinkle with flax seed meal and ground nutmeg to serve.

Fig Smoothie with Cinnamon

Preparation time: 10 minutes

Ingredients (for two servings)
6 teaspoon Greek yoghurt
1 large ripe fig
1 cup orange, apple or pineapple juice
6 teaspoon porridge oats
½ teaspoon ground cinnamon
4 ice cubes

Preparation
Wash and pat dry the figs and then chop roughly. Reserve a little to top the smoothie. Place all ingredients in a blender. Top with a teaspoon of the yoghurt, some more ground cinnamon and chopped fig.

Cucumber Sandwiches with Hummus and Mozzarella

Preparation time: 6 minutes

Ingredients
5 teaspoons hummus
10 round slices English cucumber
5 small balls of mozzarella cheese

Preparation
Spread 1 teaspoon hummus on a cucumber slice and top with a second cucumber slice. Cut Mozzarella balls in half and add to the top of the sandwich. Repeat to make 5 sandwiches.

Feta, Hummus and Bell Pepper Crackers

Preparation time: 8 minutes

Ingredients
1 large crispbread
2 tablespoons crumbled feta cheese
2 tablespoons hummus
2 tablespoons diced bell pepper

Preparation
Spread hummus on crispbread. Top with feta cheese and bell pepper.

Pistachio and Date Bites

Preparation time: 9 minutes

Ingredients (for ten servings)
2 cups pitted whole dates
1 cup raw unsalted shelled pistachios
1 cup golden raisins
1 teaspoon ground fennel seeds
¼ teaspoon ground pepper

Preparation
Combine pistachios, dates, pepper, raisins, and fennel in a food processor. Process until finely chopped. Form into about 30 balls, using about 1 tablespoon each.

Greek Cucumber Roll Ups

Preparation time: 9 minutes

Ingredients (for six servings)
1 large and cucumber
6 tablespoons roasted chopped red pepper
6 tablespoons crumbled feta
1/8 teaspoon ground black pepper
6 tablespoons roasted garlic hummus

Preparation
Use a vegetable peeler to shave off long, thin slices of cucumber. You could also cut the cucumber into thin slices using a knife. Don't use the inner slices of cucumber that are full of seeds. You should get around 10-13 useable slices off of one cucumber.

Sprinkle each slice of cucumber with a pinch of black pepper. Evenly spread about 1 1/2 teaspoon of hummus on each cucumber slice. Sprinkle 1 1/2 teaspoon of chopped red pepper and 1 1/2 teaspoon of crumbled feta on each slice.

Pick up one end of the cucumber slice and roll the cucumber around the filling. End with the seam on bottom and secure with a toothpick. Don't try to roll them up too tight or the filling will squeeze out.

Fruit and Nut Snack Mix

Preparation time: 23 minutes

Ingredients
2 cups old-fashioned oats
½ cup each of almonds, dried banana chips, tropical fruit mix, and raisins
1 tablespoon butter
¼ cup honey
1 teaspoon almond extract
1 teaspoon ground cinnamon

Preparation
Preheat oven to 350 degrees. In a saucepan, melt butter. Add honey, cinnamon, and almond extract. Mix well. Add oats and stir.

Prepare a baking pan by lining it with parchment paper.
Transfer the sticky oat mixture to the baking pan and spread it evenly. It should be no more than about 1 inch thick.

Bake for 9-10 minutes. Stir in almonds and bake for 5 minutes. Remove from oven. Add the bananas, fruits, and raisins. Cool completely before serving.

Greek Dip

Preparation time: 5 minutes

Ingredients
1 cup of plain low-fat Greek yogurt
2 grated and drained cucumbers
2 cloves minced garlic
1 tablespoon olive oil
Salt and pepper

Preparation
Mix olive oil and garlic in a bowl. Add all the remaining ingredients. Serve with broccoli, carrots, asparagus, and other vegetables.

Sweet and Sour Cream Spread with Vegetables and Fruits

Preparation time: 7 minutes

Ingredients
1/2 cup fat-free sour cream
15 cherry tomatoes
1-2 packets Sweet 'N or similar
1/4 teaspoon vanilla extract
1 one-half cups sliced fresh strawberries

Preparation
Mix the sour cream with the sweetener and vanilla extract. Serve with the strawberries and cherry tomatoes as a dipping.

Desserts

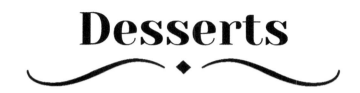

Banana Fritters with Cinnamon

Preparation time: 23 minutes

Ingredients (for four servings)
3 bananas, cut diagonally into
1 cup self-rising flour
1 beaten egg
3/4 cup sparkling water
2 teaspoon ground cinnamon sunflower oil
4 pieces each powdered sugar

Preparation
Sift flour and cinnamon into a bowl and make a well in the center. Add egg and enough sparkling water to mix to a smooth batter. Heat oil in a saucepan, enough to cover the base by 1-2 inch, so when a little batter dropped into the oil sizzles and rises to the surface. Dip banana pieces into the batter, then fry for 2-3 minutes or until golden. Remove with a slotted spoon and drain on paper towels. Sprinkle with sugar and serve hot.

Lemon Cake

Preparation time: 18 minutes

Ingredients (for eleven servings)
4 eggs
1/2 cup milk
1 cup sugar
1/2 cup sunflower oil
2 cups flour
1 tablespoon baking powder
1/2 teaspoon salt
2 tablespoon fresh lemon juice
2 tablespoon lemon zest
1/2 teaspoon vanilla extract

Preparation
Whisk eggs and sugar until light and creamy. Gently add in the flour, sunflower oil, flour, baking powder, salt, and milk. Beat until smooth, then add in vanilla and lemon juice and zest.

Pour the batter into a prepared 10 inch tube pan and bake in a preheated to 350 F oven for about 40 minutes, or until a toothpick comes out clean. Set aside to cool then turn onto a wire rack to finish cooling.

A-HA (Almond, Honey Avocado) Pudding

Preparation time: 10 minutes

Ingredients (for two servings)
2 tablespoon chopped almonds
1 ripe avocado
2 tablespoon honey
2 teaspoon vanilla extract
½ cup yogurt

Preparation
Place the avocado, honey, yogurt, and vanilla in the bowl of a food processor. Process until a smooth pudding is achieved.

Portion pudding into cups or ramekins and top with sliced almonds.

Caramelized Peaches with Goat Cheese

Preparation time: 19 minutes

Ingredients (for four servings)
2 halved peaches
2 tablespoons soft goat cheese
2 tablespoon sliced almonds
1 tablespoon honey

Preparation
Turn the oven broiler on high. Place peaches on a baking sheet, drizzle with honey and broil for 10-15 minutes, until caramelized.

Remove peaches from the oven. Place a dollop of the goat cheese on top of each apricot, followed by the almonds and then drizzle with honey. Serve warm.

Tiramisu Rice Pudding

Preparation time: 10 minutes

Ingredients (for two servings)
1½ cups cooked brown rice
1 cup milk
1 tablespoon honey
1 tablespoon cocoa powder
1 tablespoon instant coffee powder
Pinch sea salt

Preparation
In a saucepan, combine sea salt, rice, cocoa and coffee powder mixing well. Add milk and bring to a simmer on medium heat, cooking for 5 minutes.

Remove from heat and divide into two bowls, top with extra milk, cocoa powder and honey.

Blueberry Coconut Bars

Preparation time: 30 minutes

Ingredients (for five servings)
2 cups blueberries
2 cups sweetened coconut
¼ cup maple syrup
2 teaspoon ground vanilla beans

Preparation
Place all of the ingredients in your food processor and mix until smooth. Line a square baking dish with parchment paper, extending it over the sides. Pour the mixture into the baking dish and spread it evenly. Gently press the mixture down using the extended sides of the parchment paper. Refrigerate for at least 25 minutes, then slice and serve.

White Trash Bars

Preparation time: 26 minutes

Ingredients (for three servings)
1 (14-ounce) can sweetened condensed milk
1 tub French vanilla icing
1 box Ritz crackers
1 bag of toffee bits

Preparation
Preheat oven to 350 degrees F. Crush up the Ritz crackers and place them in a greased 8 x 8-inch pan.

Pour the sweetened condensed milk and toffee bits over the cracker layer. Stir it all together and pat it down into the pan. Bake for up to 20 minutes or until edges start to bubble and caramelize. Allow to cool and spread the icing on top. Cut into bars and serve.

Skillet Apples

Preparation time: 15 minutes

Ingredients (for five servings)
8 peeled and cored apples, cut into small chunks
1/8 teaspoon cloves
1/8 teaspoon nutmeg
¼ cup brown sugar
1 juiced lemon
3 tablespoons unsalted butter
1 ½ teaspoons cinnamon
1 teaspoon vanilla extract
Salt to taste

Preparation
In a large skillet or a medium cast iron skillet, melt the butter over medium heat. Add the chopped apples and the lemon juice and cook for 2 minutes. Add the cinnamon, brown sugar, vanilla, cloves, nutmeg and salt. Stir to combine, making sure the apples are fully coated. Continue to sauté over medium heat for 8-10 minutes, or until the apples are tender.

Serve warm with vanilla ice cream (or other) or on their own.

Cheat Meals

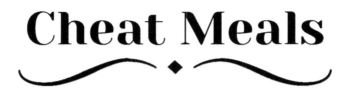

As I already mentioned, sometimes you should prepare dishes that are not with Mediterranean diet principles. This should not be too often, and you should not feel guilty about eating these dishes. There are several suggestions for these meals, while a big collection of recipes from this region is already published in my book "Ultimate Balkan Cookbook: TOP 35 Balkan dishes that you can cook right now".

Fried Breaded Zucchini *(Pohovane tikvice)*

Preparation Time: 30 minutes
Cook Time: 30 minutes

Ingredients (for four servings)
2-3 whole pieces of fresh zucchini
½ pound of bread crumbs
¼ pound of flour
2 cups of cooking oil
5 whole eggs
Salt according to taste
Dry mixed seasoning vegetables (optional)

Preparation
Peel 2-3 whole fresh pieces of zucchini and cut them endwise to thin slices, as many as you can get. Prepare two empty, deep soup plates, and pour the bread crumbs and flour into the first plate and mix them well. Break 5

whole eggs, pour them into the second plate, and whisk them well. On one side of each zucchini slice, sprinkle with salt and sprinkle the other side of the slice with a condiment, according to taste.

Roll each of the zucchini slices into the mixture of bread crumbs and flour, then roll it into the eggs, and roll it into the mixture of bread crumbs and flour. This kind of treatment gives a thicker crust after the process of frying. Meanwhile, prepare a saucepan, pour in 2 cups of cooking oil, put it onto the stove on medium, and wait for the oil to warm. Place each breaded zucchini slice into the saucepan with the hot oil. Heat the oil on medium, and when you start frying, lower the temperature down to simmer.

All sides of the zucchini slices should be fried well by turning them frequently, until they are golden brown. When the frying is complete, the fried breaded zucchini slices should be served hot, with the main meat meal (mostly with any sort of fried, breaded steaks), accompanied with French fries or mashed potatoes.

Kachamak or Palenta

Preparation Time: 30 minutes

Ingredients (for two servings)
4 cups of water
2-3 teaspoon of salt
2/3 pound corn flour (or polenta)
2 oz butter (optional)

Preparation
Bring the water to the boil in a large, heavy-based saucepan over high heat. Use a wire balloon whisk to stir the water. Gradually add the polenta in a thin, steady stream, whisking constantly until all the polenta is incorporated into the water (whisking ensures the polenta is dispersed through the liquid as quickly as possible). Don't add the polenta too quickly or it will turn lumpy. Reduce heat to low (cook the polenta over low heat, otherwise it will cook too quickly and you will need to add extra water). Simmer, stirring constantly with a wooden spoon, for 10 minutes or until the mixture thickens and the polenta is soft. (To test whether the polenta is soft, spoon a little of the polenta mixture onto a small plate and set aside to cool slightly.

Rub a little of the polenta mixture between 2 fingers to see if the grains have softened. If the grains are still firm, continue to cook, stirring constantly, over low heat until the polenta is soft.)

Remove from heat. Add cream and butter and stir until well combined. Season to taste. Serve immediately with milk, yoghurt, sour cream, or buttermilk over it.

Serbian Pandemonium salad *(Urnebes salata)*

Preparation Time: 20 minutes

Ingredients (for four servings)
1 pound feta cheese
½ cup sour cream
3 large cloves garlic crushed
1½ teaspoons sweet or hot paprika (or to taste)
1 - 2 teaspoons dried chili flakes (or to taste)

Preparation
Crush the feta with a fork into a puree. Stir in sour cream to combine thoroughly with the feta. Add crushed garlic, paprika, and chili flakes. Mix well to combine.

Garnish with additional paprika. Leave in the refrigerator overnight (the flavours will combine and develop during that time.)

One Last Thing

If you enjoyed this book or found it useful, I'd be very grateful if you'd post a short review on Amazon. Your support really does make a difference, and I read all the reviews personally so I can get your feedback and make this book even better.

Thanks again for your support and good luck with the Mediterranean lifestyle!

Please send me your feedback at
www.balkanfood.org